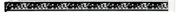

Katharine Briar-Lawson, PhD
Joan Levy Zlotnik, PhD, ACSW
Editors

Evaluation Research in Child Welfare: Improving Outcomes Through University-Public Agency Partnerships

Evaluation Research in Child Welfare: Improving Outcomes Through University-Public Agency Partnerships has been co-published simultaneously as *Journal of Health & Social Policy*, Volume 15, Numbers 3/4 2002.

Pre-publication REVIEWS, COMMENTARIES, EVALUATIONS . . .

"**T**IMELY AND IMPORTANT, particularly in its emphasis on IV-E-funded partnerships. NOT JUST FOR RESEARCHERS AND EVALUATORS . . . Even readers who do not believe they are involved in evaluation will come to appreciate the essential relationship between evaluation and program design and implementation. Answering the questions 'How can we know whether our programs are effective?' and 'How can we improve effectiveness?' requires ongoing collaborative conversations among the full range of partnership participants. This book provides a good base from which to launch such conversations."

Lois Wright, MSSW, EdD
*Assistant Dean, College of Social Work;
Director, The Center for Child
and Family Studies
University of South Carolina-Columbia*

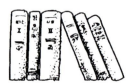

The Haworth Press, Inc.

Evaluation Research in Child Welfare: Improving Outcomes Through University-Public Agency Partnerships

Evaluation Research in Child Welfare: Improving Outcomes Through University-Public Agency Partnerships has been co-published simultaneously as *Journal of Health & Social Policy*, Volume 15, Numbers 3/4 2002.

The *Journal of Health & Social Policy* Monographic "Separates"

Below is a list of "separates," which in serials librarianship means a special issue simultaneously published as a special journal issue or double-issue *and* as a "separate" hardbound monograph. (This is a format which we also call a "DocuSerial.")

"Separates" are published because specialized libraries or professionals may wish to purchase a specific thematic issue by itself in a format which can be separately cataloged and shelved, as opposed to purchasing the journal on an on-going basis. Faculty members may also more easily consider a "separate" for classroom adoption.

"Separates" are carefully classified separately with the major book jobbers so that the journal tie-in can be noted on new book order slips to avoid duplicate purchasing.

You may wish to visit Haworth's Website at . . .

http://www.HaworthPress.com

. . . to search our online catalog for complete tables of contents of these separates and related publications.

You may also call 1-800-HAWORTH (outside US/Canada: 607-722-5857), or Fax 1-800-895-0582 (outside US/Canada: 607-771-0012), or e-mail at:

getinfo@haworthpressinc.com

Evaluation Research in Child Welfare: Improving Outcomes Through University-Public Agency Partnerships, edited by Katharine Briar-Lawson, PhD, and Joan Levy Zlotnik, PhD, ACSW (Vol. 15, No. 3/4, 2002). *"TIMELY AND IMPORTANT, particularly in its emphasis on IV-E- funded partnerships. NOT JUST FOR RESEARCHERS AND EVALUATORS. . . . Even readers who do not believe they are involved in evaluation will come to appreciate the essential relationship between evaluation and program design and implementation. Answering the questions 'How can we know whether our programs are effective?' and 'how can we improve effectiveness?' requires ongoing collaborative conversations among the full range of partnership participants. This book provides a good base from which to launch such conversations." (Lois Wright, MSSW, EdD, Assistant Dean, College of Social Work; Director, The Center for Child and Family Studies, University of South Carolina-Columbia)*

African-American Adolescents in the Urban Community: Social Services Policy and Practice Interventions, edited by Judith L. Rozie-Battle, MSW, JD (Vol. 15, No. 2, 2002). *"A comprehensive view of the challenges and opportunities that African-American youth face in today's changing society. . . . Shows that today's African-American youth face challenges that previous generations did not encounter. A must read." (Michael Bonds, PhD, Assistant Professor, Department of Educational Policy and Community Studies, University of Wisconsin-Milwaukee)*

Health and the American Indian, edited by Priscilla A. Day, MSW, and Hilary N. Weaver, DSW (Vol. 10, No. 4, 1999). *Discusses the health and mental health of Native American Indians from several aspects.*

Reason and Rationality in Health and Human Services Delivery, edited by John T. Pardeck, PhD, ACSW, Charles F. Longino, Jr., PhD, and John W. Murphy, PhD (Vol. 9, No. 4, 1998). *"A variety of perspectives that successfully challenge the pillars of modern medicine. . . . This book should be required of all health care professionals, especially those training to become physicians." (Roland Meinert, PhD, President, Missouri Association for Social Welfare, Jefferson City, Missouri)*

Selected Practical Problems in Health and Social Research, edited by Thomas E. Dinero, PhD (Vol. 8, No. 1, 1996). *"Explores some of the theoretical ideas underlying classical and modern measurement theory. These ideas form a set of guidelines for researchers, health professionals, and students in the social, psychological, or health sciences who are planning and evaluating a measurement activity." (Inquiry)*

Psychosocial Aspects of Sickle Cell Disease: Past, Present, and Future Directions of Research, edited by Kermit B. Nash, PhD (Vol. 5, No. 3/4, 1994). *"An excellent contribution to a neglected area of study and practice. . . . Offer[s] tools and techniques that one can easily incorporate into* *practice. Novice readers as well as seasoned practitioners will find the practicality of the book extremely helpful." (Social Work in Health Care)*

Health Care for the Poor and Uninsured: Strategies That Work, edited by Nellie P. Tate, PhD, and Kevin T. Kavanagh, MD, MS (Vol. 3, No. 4, 1992). *"Chapters are short and to the point with clearly defined goals, methods, techniques, and impacts and include easy-to-comprehend charts and statistics. This book will prove useful in understanding activities that may soon be an integral part of the American health care system." (Journal of Community Health)*

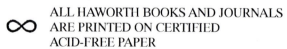

Evaluation Research in Child Welfare: Improving Outcomes Through University-Public Agency Partnerships

Katharine Briar-Lawson, PhD
Joan Levy Zlotnik, PhD, ACSW
Editors

Evaluation Research in Child Welfare: Improving Outcomes Through University-Public Agency Partnerships has been co-published simultaneously as *Journal of Health & Social Policy*, Volume 15, Numbers 3/4 2002.

The Haworth Press, Inc.
New York • London • Oxford

Evaluation Research in Child Welfare: Improving Outcomes Through University-Public Agency Partnerships has been co-published simultaneously as *Journal of Health & Social Policy™*, Volume 15, Numbers 3/4 2002.

Cover design by Jennifer M. Gaska

Library of Congress Cataloging-in-Publication Data

Evaluation research in child welfare / Katharine Briar-Lawson, Joan Levy Zlotnik, editors.
        p. cm.
    "Co-published simultaneously as Journal of health & social policy, Volume 15, Numbers 3/4 2002."
    Includes bibliographical references and index.
    ISBN 0-7890-2002-5 (hard : alk. paper) – ISBN 0-7890-2003-3 (pbk : alk. paper)
    1. Child welfare–Evaluation. 2. Evaluation research (Social action programs) I. Briar-Lawson, Katharine. II. Zlotnik, Joan Levy. III. Journal of health & social policy.
HV713 E83 2002
362.7–dc21

                                                                              2002014182

Indexing, Abstracting & Website/Internet Coverage

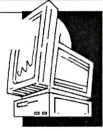

This section provides you with a list of major indexing & abstracting services. That is to say, each service began covering this periodical during the year noted in the right column. Most Websites which are listed below have indicated that they will either post, disseminate, compile, archive, cite or alert their own Website users with research-based content from this work. (This list is as current as the copyright date of this publication.)

(continued)

(continued)

Special Bibliographic Notes related to special journal issues (separates) and indexing/abstracting:

- indexing/abstracting services in this list will also cover material in any "separate" that is co-published simultaneously with Haworth's special thematic journal issue or DocuSerial. Indexing/abstracting usually covers material at the article/chapter level.
- monographic co-editions are intended for either non-subscribers or libraries which intend to purchase a second copy for their circulating collections.
- monographic co-editions are reported to all jobbers/wholesalers/approval plans. The source journal is listed as the "series" to assist the prevention of duplicate purchasing in the same manner utilized for books-in-series.
- to facilitate user/access services all indexing/abstracting services are encouraged to utilize the co-indexing entry note indicated at the bottom of the first page of each article/chapter/contribution.
- this is intended to assist a library user of any reference tool (whether print, electronic, online, or CD-ROM) to locate the monographic version if the library has purchased this version but not a subscription to the source journal.
- individual articles/chapters in any Haworth publication are also available through the Haworth Document Delivery Service (HDDS).

ABOUT THE EDITORS

Katharine Briar-Lawson, PhD, is Dean of the School of Social Welfare at the University at Albany, State University of New York. Previously, at the University of Utah, she served as Associate Dean for Research and Doctoral Studies and was a co-facilitator of four intermountain west child welfare initiatives. While at the University of Utah, Dr. Briar-Lawson directed the Social Research Institute. Prior to that, she served at Florida International University as Founder and Director of the Institute for Children and Families at Risk. She is a lead author of *Family Centered Policies and Practices: International Implications* and co-editor of *New Century Child Welfare Practice Servicing Vulnerable Children and Families.* Dr. Briar-Lawson has spearheaded university-community partnerships and family interprofessional collaboration in over 40 states. She has also served as Assistant Secretary for Children, Youth, and Families in the State of Washington.

Joan Levy Zlotnik, PhD, ACSW, has served as Executive Director of the Institute for the Advancement of Social Work Research (IASWR) since September 2000. From 1995-2000 she served as Director of Special Projects and Special Assistant to the Executive Director at the Council on Social Work Education. From 1987-1994, Dr. Zlotnik worked as Staff Director for the Commission on Families and as Government Relations Associate at the National Association of Social Workers. Previously, she held key program development and management positions in child welfare and developmental disabilities in both the private and public sectors. She has served as an adjunct faculty member and field instructor for BSW and MSW programs. For four years she was the editor of Partnerships for Child Welfare, a newsletter that highlighted cross-organizational collaborations and organized several conferences and technical meetings to promote innovation and the diffusion of effective models. She has been a consultant to federal and university projects in this area and has written about child welfare competencies and the links between child welfare and social work. She is the author of more than 18 monographs, technical assistance documents, and scholarly publications.

Evaluation Research in Child Welfare: Improving Outcomes Through University-Public Agency Partnerships

CONTENTS

EDITORIAL

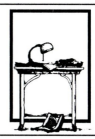

Child abuse and neglect have long been seen as health issues. The health correlates and consequences of child abuse and neglect include victim trauma and if untreated, a chain of effects, including reduced longevity, mental health challenges and high-risk behaviors, including alcohol and substance abuse, violent interactions in adulthood (Felitti & Anda et al., 1998). Horrific child abuse and neglect cases often galvanize the public into renewed concern about protecting children. These cases have led to allegations that the public child welfare systems serving children and their families are failing them. Over thirty states and large county jurisdictions have had class action lawsuits filed against them.

One of the often noted sources of failure is the absence of trained social workers. A Booz-Allen and Hamilton study, undertaken in 1987, showed that trained social workers were better prepared to produce more effective outcomes in child welfare than those with other degrees. At the same time, only an estimated 3-28% of the public child welfare workforce comprised trained social workers.

How children and families fare, once their vulnerability is recognized, has long been a social work issue. Many social work leaders as well as public child welfare administrators have abhorred the fact that the most vulnerable children and families are not only served by non-social workers, but are often served by people who may not even have a related human service degree or a baccalaureate degree of any kind. Rising drug problems such as crack and cocaine addic-

[Haworth co-indexing entry note]: "Editorial." Briar-Lawson, Katharine, and Joan Levy Zlotnik. Co-published simultaneously in *Journal of Health & Social Policy* (The Haworth Press, Inc.) Vol. 15, No. 3/4, 2002, pp. 1-3; and: *Evaluation Research in Child Welfare: Improving Outcomes Through University-Public Agency Partnerships* (ed: Katharine Briar-Lawson, and Joan Levy Zlotnik) The Haworth Press, Inc., 2002, pp. 1-3. Single or multiple copies of this article are available for a fee from The Haworth Document Delivery Service [1-800-HAWORTH, 9:00 a.m. - 5:00 p.m. (EST). E-mail address: getinfo@haworthpressinc.com].

1

tion along with co-occurring challenges such as poverty, domestic violence and mental health issues have helped to reinforce the need to have most effective services delivered by the most well prepared staff. Moreover, such challenges compel the most relevant, scientifically based approaches requiring a closer connection of public child welfare systems to social work education programs and related academic disciplines. Placing unprepared staff to protect the most vulnerable children and to address risk factors affecting the most complex and challenged families may be like having patients undergo complicated surgery without a physician and without the most up to date research knowledge about effective surgical approaches.

As a result, a social work effort to promote workforce development and to promote professional social work practice in public child welfare began in 1987. The articles featured in this volume serve as progress markers for this reprofessionalization initiative. They constitute evaluative snapshots of some of the current workforce development, including social work based education, training and capacity building in public child welfare. They also reflect social work-public child welfare partnerships and the lessons that are being learned when the research, educational and service rich resources of Schools of Social Work are harnessed to build a more well trained workforce and improved services.

As the Zlotnik article details, preparing social workers to work in public child welfare has been an historic undertaking in the field of social work and in public child welfare agencies. She sketches how NASW and collaborating national organizations such as the National Association of Public Child Welfare Administrators set out to launch a campaign to reprofessionalize child welfare practice. She notes how social work partnerships with the US Children's Bureau, access to Title IV-E funds and increases in 426 funds helped to spur this workforce development agenda.

Wehrmann, Shin and Poertner address the critical question of "training transfer." Retention and related career outcomes of trained social workers have been a critical concern in the reprofessionalization effort. Articles by Jones, Robin and Hollister, Gansle and Ellett, Dickinson and Perry, Brown, Chavkin and Peterson create a helpful database on retention. A school's research arm can serve as a capacity builder using data to foster systems and training related changes. The article by Kopels, Carter-Black and Poertner reveals how a School of Social Work's research laboratory, in partnership with the child welfare agency, has addressed the endemic community conflicts inherent in service delivery in child welfare. Anderson-Butcher, Lawson and Barkdull present evaluative data on ways that design teams have been used to foster more collaborative professional and parent-led frontline practice reforms among diverse service providers.

Training may be used to solve a problem that is not a training issue alone. Belanger's article describes how the use of cultural competence training became a tool to bring to the forefront the role of poverty as a core root cause issue for the disproportionate numbers of African American children in the public child welfare system. As delineated in the article by Ortega and Levy, complex training and educational challenges grow in the expanding managed care and privatized environments. The summary article by Smith suggests future directions for research and evaluation. It sets the stage for 21st century workforce enhancement and new developmental milestones.

Many questions for the future remain. These include the role of education, training and research in creating more effective paradigms involving services, such as mental health, welfare, substance abuse, and domestic violence as interdependent learning systems with public child welfare. Some of these may involve field units of trainees as incubators of innovative practice models and service improvements. Cross systems work teams of the future may function more like inventive, self-correcting, data driven learning systems. On the other hand, much has transpired that has created a foundation for the next round of data and evaluation-guided changes in educational preparation, service delivery, work conditions and partnerships themselves. Workforce development in public child welfare is now an integral educational agenda in social work; it is also a public good. It has in essence become a capacity building tool and a way to harness the educational, research and service related resources of schools of social work.

Katharine Briar-Lawson, PhD
Dean and Professor
School of Social Welfare
University at Albany
State University of New York

Joan Levy Zlotnik, PhD, ACSW
Executive Director
Institute for the Advancement
of Social Work Research

REFERENCES

Booz-Allen & Hamilton, Inc. (1987). The Maryland social services job analysis and personnel qualifications study, executive summary. Baltimore, Maryland, Department of Human Resources.

Felitti, V. Anda, R., Nordenberg, D. Williamson, D. Spits, A., Edwards,V., Koss, M., & Marks, J. (1998). Relationship of childhood abuse and household dysfunction to many of the leading causes of deaths in adults. *American Journal of Preventive Medicine*, 14 (4) 245-258.

Preparing Social Workers for Child Welfare Practice: Lessons from an Historical Review of the Literature

Joan Levy Zlotnik, PhD, ACSW

SUMMARY. Spurred on by national and local forces, there are currently an array of strategies underway between social work education programs and public child welfare agencies to educate current and future workers, improve agency working conditions and to develop competency-based education. These partnership efforts are frequently funded by Title IV-E and Title IV-B 426 funds. Although the majority of these efforts began in the last decade, they build on the historic connection between social work and child welfare. This connection had been weakened in the 1980s, but concerns about the need for a competent workforce and new policy and practice challenges have reinvigorated this linkage. This article examines federal support for preparing social workers in child welfare. It includes insights from almost forty years of dialogue between the education and service delivery communities on the struggle to create successful partnerships and the ongoing challenges of preparing social workers for child welfare practice. *[Article copies available for a fee from The Haworth Document Delivery Service:*

Joan Levy Zlotnik is Executive Director, Institute for the Advancement of Social Work Research, 750 First Street NE, Suite 700, Washington, DC 20002-4241 (E-mail: jzlotnik@naswdc.org).

[Haworth co-indexing entry note]: "Preparing Social Workers for Child Welfare Practice: Lessons from an Historical Review of the Literature." Zlotnik, Joan Levy. Co-published simultaneously in *Journal of Health & Social Policy* (The Haworth Press, Inc.) Vol. 15, No. 3/4, 2002, pp. 5-21; and: *Evaluation Research in Child Welfare: Improving Outcomes Through University-Public Agency Partnerships* (ed: Katharine Briar-Lawson, and Joan Levy Zlotnik) The Haworth Press, Inc., 2002, pp. 5-21. Single or multiple copies of this article are available for a fee from The Haworth Document Delivery Service [1-800-HAWORTH, 9:00 a.m. - 5:00 p.m. (EST). E-mail address: getinfo@haworthpressinc.com].

5

1-800-HAWORTH. E-mail address: <getinfo@haworthpressinc.com> Website: <http://www.HaworthPress.com> © 2002 by The Haworth Press, Inc. All rights reserved.]

KEYWORDS. Social work, child welfare, social work education, federal policy, training

   The social work profession and child welfare have an historic connection (CWLA, 1982). However, poor working environments, declassification of positions, high caseloads, increased interest by social workers in private practice or other fields of practice, and a lack of agency- and community-based resources to deal with multiple-problem families led many professionally-trained social workers away from the child welfare field (Pecora, Briar & Zlotnik, 1989). A renewed focus on the importance of a social work degree for public child welfare began in the late 1980s in response to class action lawsuits (APWA, 1991; Samantrai, 1991) and agencies challenged to provide quality services to vulnerable children and families. New collaborative efforts were undertaken to re-link social work and child welfare. These linkages were further encouraged by the passage of the Adoption and Safe Families Act of 1997 (P.L. 105-89) and the recent move by many public child welfare agencies to seek accreditation through the Council on Accreditation of Services for Families and Children (McDonald & McCarthy, 1999).
   It is estimated that in more than 40 state child welfare agencies and social work education programs are using Title IV-E funds to foster these collaborations. The funds are used to encourage social work students to pursue child welfare careers and to provide current child welfare workers with opportunities to obtain an MSW degree. Title IV-E funds are used to enhance social work education curricula, provide stipends and other supports to students, and cover the costs of field supervisors and field liaisons among other expenses (Zlotnik & Cornelius, 2000). Title IV-E is entitlement funding, created by the Child Welfare and Adoption Assistance Act of 1980 (P.L. 96-272) providing funds to states to train public child welfare staff or those preparing for employment in those agencies (GAO, 1993). Funds can be provided through state child welfare agencies to universities for "curriculum development, classroom instruction, field instruction, or any combination of these that is directly related to the agency's program. Title IV-E provides funds to cover an array of educational supports, including: faculty, stipends or on-going salaries for employees while receiving their degrees, leave costs, replacement staff for employees on educational leave, field work instructors, evaluation of field units

and curriculum, program coordinator, educational materials, books, supplies, tuition, travel, and stipends of students being recruited to work in public child welfare services (Schmid, Briar, Harris & Logan, 1993).

Concerns are raised that this child welfare/social work re-connection might retreat if the funding source was no longer available. To develop strategies that will institutionalize the connections between social work and child welfare, and especially the child welfare focused course work and field placements in BSW and MSW programs it might be useful to learn from previous efforts to promote collaboration between social work education and child welfare agencies. Examining the history of federal support for child welfare training may have important lessons for maintaining this connection for the future.

HISTORIC PRECEDENCE

Federal Support

While many perceive these partnerships to be new, this type of collaboration has a history that goes back more than 60 years. Since the 1935 inception of federally supported child welfare services, the Children's Bureau encouraged states to use child welfare services funds to provide educational leave for workers to get a social work degree (DHEW, 1965). The Title IV-B Section 426 program was created in 1962 as a response to a perceived workforce shortage for graduate level social workers who would be prepared to and interested in working in public child welfare. Section 426 was funded at $3.6 million in 1965, creating field work opportunities, traineeships and doctoral stipends in over 30 states (DHEW, 1965). It was estimated that there was a need for 10,000 graduate level social workers in child welfare, an increase of almost 50%, between 1958 and 1970 (DHEW, 1959).

The 1962 Social Security amendments created an expanded role for public social service agencies beyond financial assistance. Due to these legislative changes the Department of Health, Education and Welfare (DHEW) created a task force which made recommendations on the future social service workforce. *Closing the Gap in Social Work Manpower* (DHEW, 1965) reports that lines are not always clear between those tasks which should be assigned to social workers with graduate degrees and those tasks which can best be done by those with undergraduate degrees. This continues to be a dilemma today (Harris, 1996; NAPCWA, 1991; NASW, 1989; Zlotnik, 1993). The report also states that "inequities in salary, and unfavorable working conditions, including lack of autonomy in practice for the experienced, qualified social worker had a negative impact on recruitment and retention" (DHEW, 1965). These findings continue also to be valid (Pecora et al., 1989; Rome, 1997; Leighninger &

Ellett, 1998). Recent reports from California and Maryland continue to indicate the need for an increased number of child welfare workers in order to make the child welfare caseloads manageable (NASW-MD, 2000; SEIU, 2000).

Closing the Gap recommended that the supply of social workers be tripled through increased federal support for building expansion, faculty enlargement, and increase in scholarships and other types of financial aid, including loan forgiveness. Loan forgiveness continues to be a strategy to be pursued although it has some limitations (Rome, 1997). Implementing these recommendations resulted in federal support for the expansion of undergraduate social work education to prepare workers in the new child and family services created by the 1962 Amendments and to create a pool of students who would move on to graduate education. To respond to the perceived workforce needs in public social services, Congress included Section 707 in the 1967 Social Security Amendments, the same amendments that separated income maintenance from family welfare activities in public social service agencies (Austin, et al., 1996). Section 707 provided $3 million the first year and $5 million for the subsequent three years. The funds provided grants to colleges and universities to assist with the costs of developing, expanding, or improving undergraduate and graduate training of professional social work personnel. At least one half of the money each year was to be used for undergraduate programs, resulting in a major expansion of undergraduate social work education and expansion of social work in historically black colleges. Several other social work education programs received funds for programs that had a special minority emphasis. Even though funding for Section 707 lasted only until 1974, it had a significant impact on building social work education and bringing new social workers into public sector practice. Austin et al. (1996) suggest that Title IV-E might be the next major federal investment in social work after Section 707.

Leadership from National Organizations

Along with the Federal government's leadership on social work manpower issues, national organizations also supported the preparation of professionally trained social workers for public child welfare practice. An American Public Welfare Association (now the American Public Human Services Association) resolution on the "Goals for Meeting Social Work Manpower Needs in Public Welfare Agencies," (APWA, 1963) included (1) Clear definition of tasks which are performed by persons with professional social work education, those with a college degree and agency training, and persons with other educational backgrounds and skills; (2) Assessing skills and abilities of staff in order that they be used most effectively; (3) Recruitment of qualified applicants to meet present and future needs; (4) Establishment of a staff development program, including leave for graduate education; (5) Personnel policies which provide adequate compensation, opportunities for advancement, appropriate workloads and suitable office facilities and working conditions; and (6) Opportunities for staff to participate in administrative planning and policy formulation.

Concurrent with the implementation of the Section 426 program, a symposium sponsored by the Child Welfare League of America and Big Brothers of America addressed the implications and potential of this new child welfare training program. Representatives from APWA, social work education and state agencies addressed the challenges faced by social work students, schools of social work, and agencies in preparing students for child welfare practice. Kristenson (1964) was concerned that social work education not become dependent on grant programs since education has broader goals than just training for a specific field of practice. She also suggests that less experienced students may need more support and training from the agency because of their inexperience. Schools and agencies must plan for the individual differences of students and workers and not see all MSW graduates who enter the child welfare field as homogeneous. This was later reiterated by Gleeson, Smith and Dubos (1993) who suggested that there is no single training and preparation strategy in the development of child welfare practitioners. McCoy (1964) suggested that schools should understand the pressures agencies face and that agencies must realize that professional education has broader goals than preparation for a specific job. Baxter (1964) stresses that new workers are still learning. They bring values and knowledge to the job, but it is only in the agency that they begin to put this into practice.

The issues from this meeting were echoed over 20 years later when, in 1986, the National Association of Social Workers (NASW) hosted a meeting that brought together representatives of social work education and public child welfare agencies to address the reasons social workers are not going into public child welfare and to make recommendations to address these. Recommendations from that meeting were made in the areas of professional leadership, agency working environment, directions for professional social work education and public relations (University of Southern Maine, 1987). They are also echoed in *New Partnerships* (Briar, Hansen, & Harris, 1992), the proceedings of a 1991 symposium, funded by the U.S. Children's Bureau and hosted by Florida International University with the collaboration of several national organizations. This meeting served as a major catalyst in the re-energizing of commitments to social work education for public agency staff. A series of conferences, collaborative endeavors among national organizations and the publication of several technical assistance documents helped to promote the development of social work education/child welfare agency partnerships to address staffing issues and to improve service delivery.

A landmark in 2000 occurred when the Children's Bureau sponsored a major conference on child welfare training partnerships. The conference, co-sponsored by the Council on Social Work Education (CSWE), NASW, CWLA and the National Association of Public Child Welfare Agencies (NAPCWA) (an APHSA affiliate) highlighted the benefits achieved through child welfare partnerships. It also addressed many of the same issues raised almost 40 years earlier–recruitment and retention, BSW/MSW differentiation, and the need for multi-faceted training strategies. It also addressed the need to sustain partnerships beyond dependence on Title IV-E training funds. There was a recognition that over the past 60 years collaboration and a commitment to social work training for child welfare staff has been cyclical.

Shrinking Commitment to Social Work

The 1960s funding incentives to create a social work workforce for public human services resulted in only a small portion of the total work force receiving social work degrees. There never was a commitment to fully professionalize the workforce, nor was the profession fully committed to public sector work. The 1967 Social Security Amendments and the Social Service Block Grant legislation of 1974 encouraged contracting with private, non-profit agencies and moved many social services jobs requiring master's degree level skills out of the public sector (Gibelman, 1983). Privatization continues to be a strategy in the delivery of child welfare services today. Public agencies are identifying strategies to ensure that both the public and private agencies meet standards and have a quality workforce.

Declassification

The 1970s and 1980s saw a movement away from a commitment to have professionally trained staff. Russell (1987) found that 12% of the states had an MSW requirement in 1975, but none did in 1986. Furthermore, 16% of the states did not require a degree of any kind in 1975, while 48% did not require a degree of any kind in 1986. Declassification distanced both the social work profession and social work education from public agencies. Trends leading to declassification efforts included shortages of trained social work personnel; services integration–which, by combining a variety of social services, often made it difficult to define the tasks that should be specifically performed by a trained social worker; job mobility opportunities for workers without degrees; affirmative action; fiscal austerity; competition among related disciplines in a tight job market; and, the perceived ineffectiveness of public social services, which owing primarily to a lack of clear outcomes, stigmatized the profession–social work–most attached to the delivery of those services (NASW, 1984).

Legislative Initiatives

Growing concerns about the increasing numbers of children lingering in foster care led to the passage of the Child Welfare and Adoption Assistance Act of 1980 (Public Law 96-272). Some hoped that this new legislation would reignite the commitment to having professionally trained staff provide public child welfare services. Unfortunately, the resources and training needed to help front line workers, supervisors and administrators understand and implement the vision and service delivery components was not provided. There were no staffing or training provisions of P.L. 96-272, and at the same time Title XX social service training was cut (Allen & Knitzer, 1983). Efforts to repeal the legislation or block grant it were unsuccessful, but funding was severely cut. Between 1979 and 1981, the Children's Bureau funded Regional Child Welfare Training Centers were valuable in providing training, technical assistance, research and support to state and local child welfare agencies. Unfortunately, they were eliminated and the Section 426 funds for child welfare training were severely cut. The Section 426 program reached a funding high of $8,150,000 in 1978. In 1982, the program was cut to $3.8 million dollars and remained at approximately that level through 1995. That was similar to the funding level in 1965 when the program began. In 1992 constant dollars this is a 75% reduction from the 1978 funding level, and a far greater reduction from its 1965 inception (GAO, 1993). Successful advocacy by the ANSWER Coalition over the course of several years in the late 1990s helped to increase the 426 training program to $7 million, where it remained in 2000.

The mechanism to use Title IV-E funds was available beginning in 1980, but not publicized to social work education programs or state agencies and was little used by schools of social work for degree education until several social work education leaders and child welfare administrators began promoting its availability around 1990.

Renewed Focus on Child Welfare Staffing

In the late 1980s the failed commitment to trained staff was coupled with rising foster care caseloads, rising rates of child abuse and neglect reports, increasing numbers of class action suits, and media attention from sensationalized child deaths due to maltreatment. This lead child welfare agencies and national organizations to seek answers to the crises the children, families and agencies faced. APWA recommended increasing community-based services to prevent child abuse and neglect, new focus on services that preserve and strengthen families prior to placement and improved crisis intervention, placement and post-placement services (APWA, 1991). NAPCWA (1987) recommended that child protective staff have at least a BSW or a related degree and ideally have an MSW or a master's degree in a closely related field. The CWLA National Commission on Family Foster Care (1991) recommended that foster care be provided by "professional social workers whose education, training, certification, caseload size and supervision provide the qualifications and opportunity to meet family foster care program goals," and encouraged collaboration between child welfare agencies and social work education programs to ensure that social work education addresses the current and anticipated needs of child welfare. This was one of many calls to foster new collaboration to provide for a better trained workforce.

The passage of the Family Preservation and Support Services Provisions of the Omnibus Budget Reconciliation Act of 1993 (Public Law 103-66) was one more catalyst in the move toward a better trained work force. There are not specific staff qualifications or training standards, but states were required to provide a staff development and training plan (*Federal Register*, 1994). The social work community was encouraged to share its expertise in creating services from a family-focused perspective, undertake research and evaluation projects, be involved in training and consultation for all levels of child welfare staff and develop family-focused curricula and field instruction opportunities within social work education (NASW, 1993). Several schools of social work received contracts from states to spearhead planning activities and NASW and social work educators participated on the state planning groups.

Responding to changing policy demands such as the implementation of the Adoption and Safe Families Act of 1997 again created impetus for child welfare partnerships. The ASFA requirements suggested that staff competencies and reasonable-sized caseloads are needed to work "quicker" and "smarter" and to implement such practices as concurrent planning and family group decision-making. In addition, states needed to meet standards for the delivery of out-of-home care services.

CURRENT STRATEGIES

Recognizing that children, families and agencies are paying a price for untrained, overburdened staff, public child welfare agencies are implementing solutions to address their staffing crises. Maryland passed House Bill 1033 which requires competency testing and sets professional standards for child welfare staff. In California, SB 2030 authorized a workforce study that found that twice as many social workers were needed to meet minimum standards and three times as many to do the job according to best practices. The American Federation of State, County, and Municipal Employees (AFSCME) reports on worker's burdens and the need for staff training.

The U.S. Children's Bureau has strengthened the Section 426 discretionary grant training program to encourage social work education programs to develop competency-based education programs to prepare new students and currently employed workers for public child welfare practice. Public child welfare agencies, social work education programs, and NASW chapters are working together to utilize Title IV-E training funds to prepare new workers for child welfare practice, to assist current workers in returning to social work schools to get BSW and MSW degrees, and to improve the quality of the inservice and preservice training provided to agency staff. Current partnerships focus on field placements; financial incentives, i.e., stipends; curriculum focused on child welfare; faculty/agency staff exchanges; and helping to plan and implement system improvements. Beyond training, states and social work education programs are also beginning to develop research partnerships (McDonald and McCarthy, 1999).

Similar to the discussions at the 1963 CWLA/Big Brothers meeting, Zlotnik (1993) identified several barriers that these collaboratives need to overcome to be successful. They include social work programs may not have a focus on the needs of high-risk families or public sector practice; faculty members may not be attracted to the challenges of developing practice applications in the less than ideal settings that public agencies offer; the needs of the agency are often specific and immediate, while the education focus is broad and is designed to increase the knowledge base; social work education is broad-based and gives students limited opportunity to gain expertise in a specialization; agencies must expect to hire workers who need additional training; agencies that do not have specific positions for MSWs or require an MSW for advancement provide little incentive to hire or retain MSWs; time and resources are needed for the agency and university to sustain commitment for the long-term; and, agencies and social work education programs need to clarify job requirements for staff with different skill and educational levels, and the differential knowledge, skills and abilities that BSW graduates and MSW graduates have for different job tasks.

Partnerships emphasize collaboration which includes developing shared goals, commitment for the long-term, trusting relationships, benefits for all collaborators and common interests and objectives (Zlotnik, 1993). At the same time that agencies have made a commitment to the education and hiring of professionally trained social workers, social work education programs are making a commitment to prepare social workers for family-focused, neighborhood-based, prevention, early intervention and out-of-home placement services. Many state and local child welfare agencies are embarked on reform efforts to create more neighborhood-based, family-focused services. In many instances these reform efforts are being done in tandem with social work educators who may also be providing programmatic and/or evaluation guidance.

Current efforts to promote professional social work practice in public child welfare agencies have several common characteristics that are often included:

a. promoting competency-based education and training strategies;
b. articulating a set of values, e.g., "family-centered practice, safety of children, permanency, respect for racial and ethnic diversity, and client empowerment" (Tourse & Weitzman, 1994);
c. following-up with students who have been prepared for child welfare practice; and
d. differential hiring of BSW and MSW graduates. BSWs are more likely to be hired as case managers and MSW graduates are more likely to be hired as intensive therapists, supervisors and program managers.

Addressing recruitment and retention problems has become a shared issue between schools and agencies. Each participant recognizes that if there is going to be a long-term commitment to qualified, competent staff to meet the needs of the most vulnerable children and families, each partner has to make changes. While schools work on curriculum issues, agencies are addressing environmental issues such as desks, office, phones, computers, cars, supervisor to staff ratios, and career ladders. There is no single solution to the staffing crisis. Wasserman (1970) found that having the requisite knowledge and skills is not enough to keep new workers in child welfare. Rycraft (1994) and Ellet and Kelley and Noble (1995) describe the need to have a "goodness of fit" between the worker and the tasks to be performed. Some workers are better at crisis work, while others might do best with more long-term in depth cases. It is important for current workers who are getting MSW degrees to have job options upon their return. Puig (1995) discussed the opportunity that new MSWs who returned to a regional office had in creating job assignments in their area of interest. Rome (1997) found that one of the disincentives identified by social work students for public child welfare practice, was that while agencies might prefer a social work graduate, they will hire anyone at the same salary, leaving little incentive for persons who have invested in a degree to take that job.

The growing numbers of students doing field placements in public child welfare agencies has provided a ready pool of new hires (Miller, Fox and Burnham, 1999). Students exposed to these agencies have learned about the range of child welfare services available and been able to pick job openings that most fit with their interests. Faculty are also changing. Rather than presenting public child welfare as a last resort for employment, current students are being encouraged to see it as a great learning ground for practice.

IMPLICATIONS

Although social work education and public child welfare are building new relationships, the connection is often tenuous. Many of the reconnections are supported by federal Title IV-E funds that may be vulnerable to federal child welfare refinancing strategies. It is critical for agency and university partners to organize advocacy, research and evaluation efforts to institutionalize these efforts over the long haul. Agencies should maintain their commitment to well-trained staff who are qualified and competent to do assessments and intervention. Universities and agencies must continue to work together to develop a long-term training strategy that invests in current workers and also prepares future workers for agency work. Universities must ensure relevant curriculum and educational strategies that provide students with a base-line for child welfare practice. Agencies must continue to focus on improving the working environments and the resources available to help make the worker's job manageable.

Will the lessons of the past be heeded? Encouraging social workers into child welfare needs to be sustained by more than funding resources. There must be commitment on the part of the agency and the university together or the professionally trained staff will not be there. Research strategies must be developed to create evidence to demonstrate for state legislatures, agency heads, governors and the media that there is a link between well-trained staff and child and family outcomes.

But hiring child welfare staff with social work degrees and lowering caseloads will not alone solve the problems of service delivery. Workplaces must be welcoming to social work graduates and must provide safe, ethically sound and resourceful places to work. Students considering child welfare must learn that it is a stressful but rewarding place to work. Agencies and universities must offer support through quality supervision and help child welfare workers learn coping strategies while in school and on the job. The profession will continue to grapple with the differentiation of BSW and MSW education and job responsibilities. The distinctions, in practice, are often related to what is available in the setting and the community rather than to specific job tasks.

As the welfare state devolves, social work education must remain involved and connected to the most vulnerable children and families. The link between child welfare and social work has gone full circle. This is a time to keep it connected through strengthening ties, rather than letting a changing social structure break the cycle.

REFERENCES

AFSCME. (1998). *Double Jeopardy: Caseworkers at Risk Helping at Risk Kids.* Washington, DC: AFSCME Public Policy Office.

Allen, M. L. & Knitzer, J. (1983). Child welfare: Examining the policy framework. In B. McGowan & W. Meezan (Eds.), *Child welfare: Current dilemmas, future directions* (pp. 93-142). Illinois: Peacock.

American Public Welfare Association. (1991). Child welfare litigation. *W-Memo.* Washington, DC: Author.

American Public Welfare Association. (1991). *Commitment to change: Report from the National Commission on Child Welfare and Family Preservation.* Washington, DC: Author.

American Public Welfare Association. (1963). Goals for meeting social work manpower needs in public welfare agencies. *Public Welfare, 21*(1), p. 2.

Baxter, E. (1964). The agency's expectations from the beginning professional worker. *Child Welfare, 43* (2), 77-79.

Briar, K., Hansen, V. & Harris, N. (Eds.). (1992). *New partnerships: Proceedings from the National Public Child Welfare Symposium.* Miami, FL: Florida International University.

Child Welfare League of America. (1982). *Child welfare as a field of social work practice* (2nd ed.). New York: Author.

Ellett, A., Kelley, B., & Noble, D. (1995, October). *Personnel needs and professionalization issues in child welfare.* Paper presented at National Association of Social Workers conference in Philadelphia, PA.

Family Preservation and Support Services Program: Proposed Rule. (1994, October 4). *Federal Register, 59* (191), 50646-50673.

General Accounting Office. (1993). *Federal policy on Title IV-E share of training costs.* Washington, DC: Author.

Gibelman, M. (1983). Social work education and the changing nature of public agency practice. *Journal of Education for Social Work, 19* (3), 21-28.

Gleeson, J., Smith, J., & Dubos, A. (1993). Developing child welfare practitioners: Avoiding the single-solution seduction. *Administration in Social Work, 17* (3), 21-37.

Harris, N. (1996). *Social work education and public human services partnerships: A technical assistance document.* Alexandria, VA: Council on Social Work Education.

Kristenson, A. (1964). The child welfare worker: Strengths and limitations in his professional training. *Child Welfare, 43* (2), 64-71.

Leighninger, L., & Ellett, A. (1998). Deprofessionalization in Child Welfare: Historical Analysis and Implications for Social Work Education. Paper presented at the CSWE Annual Program Meeting, March 7, 1998, Orlando, FL.

Lieberman, A., Russell, M., & Hornby, H. (1989). *National survey of child welfare workers.* Portland, ME: University of Southern Maine, National Resource Center for Management and Administration.

McCoy, J. (1964). Are the schools adequately training students for child welfare? *Child Welfare 43* (2), 73-75.

McDonald, J. & McCarthy, B. (1999). Effective Partnershp Models Between the State Agencies, Community, the University and Community Service Providers. In *1999 child welfare training symposium: Changing paradigms of child welfare practice: responding to opportunities and challenges*, pp. 43-73. Washington, DC: U.S. Children's Bureau.

Miller, V., Fox, S., & Burnham, D. (December, 1999). Pre-Service Certification Program Garners Praise in Kentucky. *Partnerships for Child Welfare Newsletter*, Vol. 6, #2, December 1999. Alexandria, VA: Council on Social Work Education.

National Association of Public Child Welfare Administrators. (1987). *Guidelines for a model system of protective services for abused and neglected children and their families.* Washington, DC: American Public Welfare Association.

National Association of Public Child Welfare Administrators. (1991). *Public child welfare agencies and schools of social work: The current status of collaboration.* (Available from American Public Welfare Association, 810 First St. NE, Washington, DC 20002).

National Association of Social Workers. (1993, November 19). *Family preservation and support services provisions included in the Omnibus Budget Reconciliation Act of 1993* (Government Relations Update). Washington, DC: National Association of Social Workers.

National Association of Social Workers. (1989). *The staffing crisis in child welfare: Report from a colloquium.* Silver Spring, MD: Author.

National Association of Social Workers, Florida Chapter. (1984). *Report and recommendations of the Florida chapter NASW professional standards–classification ad hoc committee.* Tallahassee, FL: Author.

National Association of Social Workers, Maryland Chapter. (November-December 2000). Recruitment, Retention of Public Child Welfare Workers, *Maryland Sentinel.*

National Commission on Family Foster Care. (1991). *A blueprint for fostering infants, children, and youths in the 1990's.* Washington, DC: Child Welfare League of America.

Pecora, P., Briar, K., & Zlotnik, J. (1989). *Addressing the program and personnel crisis in child welfare: A social work response.* Silver Spring, MD: National Association of Social Workers.

Puig, M. & Rowland, P. (1995, October). *The reprofessionalization of a public child welfare agency.* Paper presented at the National Association of Social Workers conference in Philadelphia, PA.

Rome, S. H. (1997). The child welfare choice: An analysis of social work students career plans. *Journal of Baccalaureate Social Work*, vol. 3 (1). 31-48. Rome–student loan.

Russell, M. (1987). *1987 national study of public child welfare job requirements.* Portland, ME: University of Southern Maine, National Child Welfare Resource Center for Management and Administration.

Rycraft, J. (1994). The party isn't over: The agency role in the retention of child welfare workers. *Social Work, 39* (1), 75-80.

Samantrai, K. (1991, November). Lawsuits to force governments to provide better child welfare services: The story of some states. *NASW California News* (p. 7).

Schmid, D., Briar, K., Harris, N., & Logan, J. (1993, February). Creating an interdependent services and training financing strategy. *Partnership Newsletter.* Miami, FL: Florida International University Department of Social Work, Institute for Children and Families at Risk.

SEIU Local 535. (September 2000). Social work can make a difference but workers need the time to help. (www.seiu535.org/dragonarticles/sept2000/SWAwareness.htm).

Tourse, R., & Weitzman, D. (1995, March). *Aligning field curriculum with child welfare competencies defined by school-agency partnerships.* Paper presented at the 41st Annual CSWE Annual Program Meeting.

U.S. Department of Health, Education and Welfare. (1965). *Closing the gap in social work manpower.* Washington, DC: Author.

U.S. Department of Health, Education and Welfare. (1959). *Report of the advisory council on child welfare services.* Washington, DC: Author.

University of Southern Maine. (1987). *Professional social work practice in public child welfare: An agenda for action.* Portland, ME: University of Southern Maine, Center for Research and Advanced Study.

Vinokur-Kaplan, D. (1987). Where did they go? A national follow-up of child welfare trainees. *Child Welfare, 66* (5), 411-421.

Wasserman, H. (1970). Early careers of professional social workers in a public child welfare agency. *Social Work, 15* (6), 93-101.

Weisbrod, H. (1964). Training public welfare staff to help children. *Child Welfare, 43* (2), 80-86.

Zlotnik, J. (1993). *Social work education and public human services: Developing partnerships.* Alexandria, VA: Council on Social Work Education.

Zlotnik, J. L. & Cornelius, L. (2000). Preparing social work students for child welfare careers: The use of Title IV-E training funds in social work education. *Journal of Baccalaureate Social Work*, vol. 5, #2, pp. 1-14.

APPENDIX. Social Work Education and Public Child Welfare Partnerships

HIGHLIGHTS OF A LONG HISTORY

1935 • Passage of the Child Welfare Provisions of the Social Security Act. The Children's Bureau supports states spending some funds to provide social work education for staff.

1962 • Creation of the Title IV-B, Section 426 Discretionary Training Grant Program to provide funds to institutions of higher learning to train individuals in the child welfare field. Funded at $3.5 million in 1965, this program was a major source of funding to provide social work education for agency workers and to provide opportunities for students to pursue child welfare careers.

1980 • Passage of Child Welfare and Adoption Assistance Act of 1980 (P.L. 96-272). No specific staffing qualifications were included. Created Title IV-E training which allows for state child welfare agencies to provide funds to universities for curriculum development, classroom instruction, field instruction, or any combination of these that is directly related to the agency's program–75% federal match. Includes foster and adoptive parent training and worker training, including preparing students for pubic child welfare practice. Few universities and agencies use these funds to prepare workers in the unversity.

1986-1988 • **A Staffing Crisis in Child Welfare is Identified.** Agencies were having difficulty recruiting and retaining competent, committed staff. The dilemma was that social work felt that child welfare agencies were not interested in attracting and retaining professional social workers and child welfare agencies felt that social work education was not providing the relevant education for contemporary child welfare practice. Actions began to occur.

- NASW hosts symposium on "Professional Social Work Practice in Public Child Welfare," March 1986 with support from the HHS Office of Human Development Services, creates a task force on promoting professional social work practice in public child welfare, Commission on Families makes promoting professional social work practice in public child welfare an agenda priority.

- CWLA 1988 Biennial Resolution on Recruitment and Retention of Staff creates task force and study.

- NAPCWA/APWA publication of *Guidelines for a Model System of Protective Services for Abused and Neglected Children and Their Families.*

- American Humane Association publishes guidelines for staffing child protection agencies which recommend that staff have social work degrees.

- Booz-Allen, Hamilton study in Maryland suggest that hiring staff with social work degrees is more cost effective than just providing training.

- NAPCWA forum addresses the need for partnerships between social work education and child welfare agencies to address staffing issues.

1989

- Publication of *Addressing the Program and Personnel Crisis in Public Child Welfare: A Social Work Response*, Pecora, Briar & Zlotnik, NASW.
- NASW hosts a colloquium on the staffing crisis in child welfare, including representatives from NAPCWA, CSWE, CWLA and the Children's Bureau.

1990

- U.S. Advisory Board on Child Abuse and Neglect recommends that child protective service staff meet national educational standards and that guidelines be established regarding caseloads and staff training.

1991

- Children's Bureau provides funding to Florida International University to host The National Child Welfare Training Conference which brought together 200 social work educators and agency administrators from over 40 states to address strategies to create partnerships to address issues of recruitment, retention and staff competencies. *New Partnerships*, Briar, Hansen and Harris, Florida International University, provides the proceeding from that meeting.
- Universities and agencies strengthen their collaborative efforts to provide social work education for current and future workers.

1992

- Children's Bureau funds 11, 5-year, interdisciplinary child welfare training grants to focus on competency-based education, and requiring social work programs to work in partnerships with child welfare agencies.
- Children's Bureau funds Florida International University to provide technical assistance and conferences which promote partnerships between social work education programs and public child welfare agencies.
- Ford Foundation provides a grant to CSWE–*Social Work Education and Public Human Services Partnership Project.*
- CWLA hosts a colloquium, in partnership with CSWE, on building partnerships between child welfare agencies and social work education programs and publishes *Building Partnerships: Schools and Agencies Advancing Child Welfare Practice* and *Staffing the Child Welfare Agency: Recruitment and Retention.*
- APWA, in collaboration with CSWE, hosts a forum in San Diego "Education for Service: Public Human Service Agencies and Schools of Social Work," which focused on successful collaborative efforts.

1993
- CWLA, in collaboration with NASW, CSWE, and with funding from HHS, develops "Start Me Up," a video targeted to recruit high school and college students into child welfare careers.
- CSWE publishes *Social Work Education and Public Human Services: Developing Partnerships*.
- Children's Bureau funds additional grants to social work education programs to prepare students for child welfare careers.
- NASW surveys student members to determine their interest in child welfare careers–*Choosing Child Welfare*, Rome, NASW Office of Government Relations.
- Passage of the Family Preservation and Support Provisions of P.L. 103-66. Collaboration and partnerships among agencies and between agencies and universities are encouraged to plan and implement the provisions. Several schools of social work carry out the planning task for the state and many social work educators are involved in the planning and evaluation process.

1994
- "Expanding Partnerships for Vulnerable Children, Youth and Families" conference takes place in Tysons Corner, VA, not only addressing child welfare partnerships, but also addressing the need for cross-systems and cross-university partnerships.

1996
- CSWE's Ford Project publishes *Social Work Education and Public Human Services Partnerships: A Technical Assistance Document*.
- Over the past 5 years more than 60 child welfare training grants under Section 426 have been granted to social work education programs to prepare 100's of students for child welfare careers.
- Currently more than 30 BSW programs and 40 MSW programs receive Title IV-E funds to prepare students for child welfare careers.

1997
- The Adoption and Safe Families Act is passed which reinforces the need for well-trained child welfare staff, encouraging new partnerships between child welfare and social work education program.

1999
- Children's Bureau hosts child welfare training symposium to examine the outcomes from university agency partnerships. The symposium is co-hosted by NASW, CSWE, CWLA and NAPCWA.

2000
- Children's Bureau sponsors National Child Welfare Training Conference which brings together 300 university and agency partners to learn from each others experiences in building a competent workforce and improving child welfare service delivery.

Transfer of Training:
An Evaluation Study

Kathryn Conley Wehrmann, PhD
Hyucksun Shin, MSW
John Poertner, DSW

SUMMARY. This article describes an evaluative study focused on the transfer of trained knowledge and skills back to the practice setting. A model of transfer was developed based on factors identified in the literature. Survey methodology was used to obtain data from training participants at the completion of training and again six months later. They assessed attainment of learning outcome and its other model components. The regression model that resulted accounted for 52% of the variance in participants' perceptions of their learning. Training participants having an opportunity to perform new tasks on the job, support of peers for using new skills and familiarity with the content prior to training were the variables in the model. Recommendations for training and evaluation of training efforts are also presented. *[Article copies available for a fee from The Haworth Document Delivery Service: 1-800-HAWORTH. E-mail address: <getinfo@haworthpressinc.com> Website: <http://www.HaworthPress.com> © 2002 by The Haworth Press, Inc. All rights reserved.]*

Kathryn Conley Wehrmann is affiliated with the Department of Social Work, Illinois State University, Campus Box 4650, Normal, IL 61790-4650.

Hyucksun Shin and John Poertner are affiliated with the School of Social Work, University of Illinois at Urbana-Champaign, Urbana, IL 61801.

This research was funded in part by the Illinois Department of Children and Family Services.

[Haworth co-indexing entry note]: "Transfer of Training: An Evaluation Study." Wehrmann, Kathryn Conley, Hyucksun Shin, and John Poertner. Co-published simultaneously in *Journal of Health & Social Policy* (The Haworth Press, Inc.) Vol. 15, No. 3/4, 2002, pp. 23-37; and: *Evaluation Research in Child Welfare: Improving Outcomes Through University-Public Agency Partnerships* (ed: Katharine Briar-Lawson, and Joan Levy Zlotnik) The Haworth Press, Inc., 2002, pp. 23-37. Single or multiple copies of this article are available for a fee from The Haworth Document Delivery Service [1-800-HAWORTH, 9:00 a.m. - 5:00 p.m. (EST). E-mail address: getinfo@haworthpressinc.com].

KEYWORDS. Child welfare, training, evaluation

INTRODUCTION

Given the importance attributed to training for careers in protecting children and providing them permanent homes, as well as the significant amount spent on training, it is not surprising that there is considerable interest in assessing the translation of specialized training to the field. United States child welfare services currently involve approximately 560,000 children and youth in out of home care alone (USDHHS, 2000). Title IV-E spending on training in public child welfare was $188 million for fiscal year 2000 (U.S. Government Printing Office, 1998). With states required to match a minimum of 25% in order to access Title IV-E funds, the total amount spent for child welfare training during FY 2000 is at least $250 million. This does not include the expenditures of private agencies or staff who pay their own way to continuing education workshops or advanced degrees.

Public child welfare agencies rely heavily upon training for a variety of purposes, including preparing employees to provide children safe and permanent homes. Training also serves as a primary vehicle for introducing changes brought about by new legislation and increasingly complex client situations. Training is also a means for agencies to hold employees accountable for practices within acceptable bounds.

Despite the fact that training is a major tool in an effort to develop and maintain sound practice, there is surprisingly little research on the transfer of training from the classroom to the field (Baldwin & Ford, 1988; Curry, Caplan & Knuppel, 1994; Ford, Quinones, Sego, & Sorra, 1992; Gregoire, Propp, & Poertner, 1998; Latham, 1988; Miller & Dore, 1991; Noe, 1986; Pecora, Dodson, Teather, & Whittaker, 1983; Seipel, 1986; Tannenbaum & Yukl, 1992; Tziner, Haccoun & Kadish, 1991). Most evaluations involve counting the number of people who attended training and reporting on the amount of money spent (Seipel, 1986). It is also typical for training evaluation to focus on participant opinions of the training and the methods used. To know if training is worth the investment of time and money evaluations need to focus on the transfer of knowledge and skills to the job.

An evaluation focusing on the transfer of knowledge and skills can provide insight into factors both inside and outside the training process that serve to enhance or inhibit the transfer of knowledge and skills to the workplace. Evaluation at this level can also place agencies in a more proactive position to create organizational environments where the transfer of training is enhanced. Training with the goal of preparing child welfare workers to provide services intended to bring about positive outcomes for families requires evaluation strategies that actually assess whether training has produced the intended result. The study reported here is an evaluation from the trainee's perspective of the transfer of training to the job.

REVIEW OF THE LITERATURE

The evaluation study reported on here was based upon a review of the transfer of training literature and preliminary studies conducted by Gregoire, Propp, and Poertner (1998). An initial review of this literature identified sets of variables related to the transfer of training. These include individual attributes, instructional design, and the organizational environment.

Individual Attributes. Individual attributes that influence the transfer of training include the trainee's expectations of the training event, involvement in decisions to participate in training, feelings of self-efficacy and locus of control (Noe, 1986; Tziner et al., 1991). Each of the attributes is described below.

Expectancy. Expectancy refers to the level of knowledge trainees have about the training event and what it is intended to accomplish. The more trainees know about their future training sessions such as learning goals, expected outcomes, and methods of training, the more likely that transfer of training will occur (Baldwin & Ford, 1988; Clark, Dobbins, & Ladd, 1993; Noe, 1986; Noe & Schmitt, 1986).

Decision Involvement. Decision involvement refers to the extent to which trainees are involved both in choosing training and providing input into training content (Clark et al., 1993; Guthrie & Schwoerer, 1994). Mandatory training, identified as an inhibitor to decision involvement, may affect motivation through increased resistance and contribute to a hostile or non-supportive work climate (Guthrie & Schwoerer, 1994; Pecora et al., 1983; Wright & Fraser, 1988). On the other hand, voluntary participation in training has been found to result in stronger beliefs in training significance and higher satisfaction with training outcomes.

Self-Efficacy. Self-efficacy is the belief in one's ability to successfully perform a given task (Bandura, 1986). It has been identified by many as a catalyst to behavior change and maintenance (Karl, O'Leary-Kelly & Martocchio, 1993; Latham, 1988; Noe, 1986; Tannenbaum & Yukl, 1992). Individuals who possess high levels of self-efficacy will put forth substantial effort to master new behavioral demands and work towards higher performance levels (Noe, 1986). Morin (1999) found that measures of self-efficacy were higher for individuals who engaged in mental practice activities following participation in a formal training program.

Locus of Control. Locus of control is a person's perception of the control they have over events. Individuals are assumed to fit in one of two categories, internal or external (Baldwin & Ford, 1988; Noe, 1986). Individuals who are characterized as being internals feel in control of their environment and able to influence it. In contrast, individuals characterized as externals perceive that they lack control over their environments, and may feel victimized by environmental effects (Noe, 1986; Tziner et al., 1991). The implications of locus of control theory for transfer of training is that those categorized as internals will exert more effort in training by gathering relevant information. Internals may more actively seek ways to fulfill expectancies such as promotion and recognition (Noe, 1986). Externals may not be as likely to believe that mastering the training content is within their control (Noe, 1986; Baldwin & Ford, 1988).

Instructional Design. Instructional design is another factor that is said to contribute to training transfer. An effective training curriculum is reported to include clear objectives, is relevant to the work context, and presents the content in a variety of ways. Training should use trainers who are skilled, possess credibility from the trainee's point of view, and provide performance feedback (Baldwin & Ford, 1988; Curry et al., 1994; Doucek & Austin, 1986; Ford et al., 1992; Hagen, 1990; Noe, 1986; Pecora, 1989; Rooney, 1988; Seipel, 1986; Tziner et al., 1991; Vinokur-Kaplan, 1987).

Tannenbaum and Yukl (1992) suggests that it is important for training courses to support and mirror the mission and goals of the organization in order to establish congruence between the work environment and the training material. Tziner et al. (1991) suggest that the level of training transfer may be improved by teaching underlying principles and incorporating elements such as over-learning, stimuli which mirror the work environment, and goal setting. Performance feedback may also increase self-efficacy and influence transfer of training (Clark et al., 1993).

Clark (1991) asserts that trainer credibility involves a combination of trustworthiness and expertise as perceived by the trainee. Processes that involve interaction with participants, goal setting, role-playing, behavior modeling, and performance feedback are also important (Baldwin & Ford, 1988, Tannenbaum & Yukl, 1992). Together these processes may increase the chances of training transfer (Baldwin & Ford, 1988; Curry et al., 1994; Guthrie & Schwoerer, 1994).

Organizational Environment. Organizational environment influences are both actual and perceived (Baldwin & Ford, 1988; Noe, 1986; Tziner et al., 1991). Even before training is presented, if the trainee does not perceive the work environment as being supportive, the transfer of learning is apt to be negatively affected (Noe, 1986; Tziner et al., 1991; Baldwin & Ford, 1988; Clark et al., 1993). Facets of the work environment that may influence both the actual and perceived work climate include the level and type of support from peers and supervisors, the opportunity to use skills, time to use the skills, and the role of the supervisor before and after the training (Baldwin & Ford, 1988; Ford et al., 1992).

Supervisory Support. Several researchers suggest that the supervisor may be the most important factor in the transfer of training process (Baldwin & Ford, 1988; Bowne, 1999; Gregoire, 1994; Kozlowski & Doherty, 1989; Olivero, Bane, & Kopelman, 1997; Tannenbaum & Yukl, 1992). Factors found to inhibit transfer of training included supervisors who were not prepared to listen to new ideas and allow experimentation, an overload of work, unplanned work, and difficulty in convincing older staff to make changes. Bowne (1999) found that supervisor interventions intended to increase the trainee's understanding of how training was linked to corporate goals and to help them focus on specific post-training behaviors increased the impact of training. Olivero et al. (1997) examined the effects of coaching of employees (including goal setting, collaborative problem solving, practice, feedback, and evaluation), following a training program and found that it increased productivity.

Supervisor's attitudes toward training may strongly affect the value that the employee places on training (Curry et al., 1994). Staff who perceive their supervisor as apathetic toward training are unlikely to see the relevance of the training (Garavaglia, 1993). Employees whose supervisors were not supportive or had a negative attitude toward training have also been found to have difficulty maintaining skills learned in training (Garavaglia, 1993). This suggests that the supervisory role most likely to support transfer of training is one that involves developing a supportive, rewards based environment that includes performance feedback, mentoring, modeling, and positive attitudes toward training (Curry et al., 1994; Erera & Lazar, 1993; Ford et al., 1992; Noe, 1986; Seipel, 1986; Tziner et al., 1991; Tannenbaum & Yukl, 1992; Vinokur-Kaplan, 1987; Wright & Fraser, 1988).

Peer Support. The social climate of the work environment defined as the level of support that trainees receive from peers as well as supervisors is a major factor affecting training transfer (Guthrie & Schwoerer, 1994; Kozlowski & Doherty, 1989; McDonald, 1991; Tannenbaum & Yukl, 1992; Tziner et al., 1991). Trainees are more likely to transfer what they have learned in training if they feel that peers will be supportive and patient with their efforts to transfer newly learned skills (Tziner et al., 1991). The use of "buddy systems" in which peers are paired and instructed to provide feedback and reinforcement to each other has been useful in enhancing the transfer of training (Tannenbaum & Yukl, 1992).

Opportunity to Use Skills. A trainee's opportunity to perform trained tasks on the job has a major impact on transfer of training and perceptions of training effectiveness (Ford et al., 1992). Factors hypothesized to be key influences on creating opportunities to perform include organizational structure, work context, and individual characteristics such as ability and self-efficacy. A supervisor's perceptions of a staff member's capability, skills, and likability is also related to having greater opportunity for being assigned more complex and differential tasks that enhance the likelihood of transfer (Ford et al., 1992). Supervisors are in the best position to provide opportunities for practice and performance by planning practice activities and assigning new tasks that involve the training content (Garavaglia, 1993). Bennett, Lehman and Forst (1999) found that employees who participated in a formal training event and then felt impeded from applying what they had learned in training reported lower levels of transfer than employees who perceived more supportive organizational transfer climate. Gregoire (1994) reported that workers identified the most common obstacles to implementing application of training plans as being the daily rigors of child welfare practice, refusal by supervisor to endorse proposed practice changes, limited resources, need to provide assistance to co-workers, and backlog of paper work.

METHODOLOGY

This study used a longitudinal survey design that asked training participants to assess their acquisition and use of skills at the conclusion of training and again six months later. The change in participant's views of what they learned and use is the assessment of training transfer. The self-assessment conducted six months after completing training was the dependent variable with the same assessment at the conclusion of training treated as an independent variable to assess change. These variables were constructed by identifying the learning outcomes for the training and having participants rate the acquisition and use of each of these objectives on a 6-point scale. The item responses ranged from "strongly disagree" (1) "to strongly agree" (6).

The independent variables in this study were trainee's responses on scales developed to assess individual attributes, elements of instructional design and the organizational environment.[1] The scales for each of these elements of training transfer included sub-scales reflecting the dimensions identified in the literature. These independent variables were constructed using the literature review as a guide. Most studies of this type do not use standardized scales; instead they use questionnaire items developed by the researcher. When possible, this study used items from previous research. The researchers used the concepts in the literature to write items for the other scales. All of the scales were pilot tested in a preliminary study. Items that did not contribute to the reliability of the scale were deleted or rewritten.

One additional variable was added as a result of focus groups conducted after a pilot test of the training. Trainees did not have the opportunity to select the training or its content and many reported being familiar with the content and did not find the training useful. Consequently, a content familiarity variable was added to the study.

Trainees completed one instrument at the end of the training. It asked trainees to assess their acquisition of the clinical practice learning outcomes, the instructional design and pre-training transfer factors. Trainees were asked to complete a second instrument six months later. This instrument asked them to reassess the learning outcomes as well as the post-training elements of the transfer model. In addition, participants were asked to respond to two open-ended items related to personal motivation to use skills and knowledge or other benefits of training. Demographic information such as years of experience with the agency, type of caseload, and educational background were also requested.

The 367 workers who attended training between February 1998 and the end of July 1998 received the initial survey shortly after the conclusion of training. A total of 254 (69%) of the trainees completed the survey. At the six-month follow-up, 129 participants completed the survey for a response rate of 51% of those who completed the first questionnaire.

Over 50% of respondents held degrees in psychology, sociology, social work, or criminal justice. Of the 254 participants, 125 (50%) indicated that they did not have a graduate degree. Of those reporting a graduate degree, 43 (17%) indicated that they held the MSW degree, with 8 (3%) indicating that they were working on their MSW degree. The next most frequently reported graduate degree (7) was a masters in counseling. Over 50% of respondents identified their primary agency responsibility as being either child protection or work with families where the children were at home. Another 15% reported that they had a mixed caseload, including placement and intact family cases. Nearly half of the respondents reported 4 years or less of experience with the agency with the remainder reported between 4 and 28 years of experience.

FINDINGS

The means and standard deviations for each of the scales are reported in Table 1. Participant's responses regarding attainment of the learning outcomes at the completion of training ranged from "somewhat agree" to "agree" that they had achieved the learning outcome. Most of the items (17 out of 19) had mean responses above 4.69 on a 6-point scale. Self-assessment conducted six months after training resulted in a drop in the overall dependent variable mean from 95 to 88.

TABLE 1. Clinical Practice Training Learning Outcomes and Independent Variables

	Mean	SD
Clinical Practice Training Learning Outcomes		
Learning Outcomes (Time 1)	94.8	16.8
Learning Outcomes (Time 2)	88.4	19.1
Individual Attributes		
Locus of Control	29.9	9.1
Self-Efficacy	23.9	6.2
Perceived Utility	12.5	3.8
Decision Involvement	7.9	2.5
Trainee Expectancy	7.1	2.9
Familiarity with the Content[2]	3.8	1.2
Instructional Design		
Trainer Attributes	48.8	11.4
Performance Feedback	5.2	1.1
Curriculum Design	51.7	10.7
Training Environment	3.8	1.7
Organizational Environment		
Supervisory Support Pre-Training	9.7	4.5
Supervisory Support Post-Training	22.4	8.0
Supervisor Feedback	3.9	1.6
Supervisor Provides Incentives to Use Skills	15.6	5.4
Opportunity to Use Skills	7.8	2.8
Practice and Rehearsal	7.6	2.7
Peer Support Pre-Training	13.6	6.9
Peer Support Post-Training	9.0	2.2
Work Environment	4.0	1.5

[2] This item ranged from (1) 0-19%, (2) 20-39%, (3) 40-59%, (4) 60-79%, (5) 80-100%

Correlations between the transfer of training variables and the learning outcomes assessed by trainees six months following training are reported in Table 2. Two of the individual attribute variables were strongly correlated with the self-assessment of learning outcomes. These were self-efficacy ($r = .36$, $p < .01$) and perceived utility ($r = .38$, $p < .01$). Locus of control was not significantly correlated with the dependent variable.

Of the instructional design variables only the training environment was not correlated with the learning outcomes. Trainer attributes, performance feed-

TABLE 2. Correlations Between the Independent Variables and the Dependent Variable

Individual Attributes

Locus of Control	.09
Self-Efficacy	.36***
Perceived Utility	.38***

Training Curriculum

Trainer Attributes	.44***
Feedback	.35***
Instructional Design	.42***
Training Environment	.07

Pre-Training Factors

Decision Involvement	.17*
Peer Support	.20**
Supervisor Support	.11
Trainee Expectancy	.16*

Post-Training Factors

Opportunity to Perform	.47***
Practice	.43***
Incentives	.44***
Supervisor Support	.36***
Peer Support	.40***
Work Environment	.26***
Supervisor Feedback	.27***

* Indicates significant correlation, $p < .15$
** Indicates significant correlation, $p < .05$
*** Indicates significant correlation, $p < .01$

back and curriculum design were all significantly correlated with the learning outcomes at the $p < .01$ level.

In the organizational environment only supervisor support prior to training was not correlated with learning outcomes. Peer support prior to training had a weak correlation ($p < .01$) to the dependent variable. All the other organizational environment variables were correlated with the learning outcomes at the $p < .01$ level.

The final step of the data analysis was to develop a multivariate model to identify variables that explained as much of the variance as possible in the self-assessment of the learning outcomes. Since this analysis focused on explaining respondents use of skills as measured by the change in their reporting of learning and use, learning outcome assessment at time 1 was entered into the equation first. Since this was an exploratory study, the approach developed by Dottalo (1994) was used. In this approach those variables with a significant correlation with the learning outcomes indicated by an alpha of .15 or less were included in model building. This is done so those potentially important variables are not excluded because of failure to meet the more stringent criteria of an alpha of .05 or better. Backward pair-wise linear regression was then used to develop the model that best accounted for the variance in the dependent variable. The resulting model is presented in Table 3. This set of variables accounted for 52% of the variance in workers perceptions of their learning and use of learning objectives six months after training. The model also had a significant F value of 35.15 (p < .001).

The variables that explained trainees use of trained knowledge and skills were the opportunity to perform new tasks on the job, the support of peers upon returning to the job and familiarity with the content. The relationship between familiarity with the content and the dependent variable was negative. Those participants who reported that they were most familiar with the content reported learning and using the least knowledge. This supported focus group findings following the pilot testing of the curriculum where many workers reported that they already knew the material presented in the training. This is not surprising since an outside contractor designed this training and all workers were required to participate. The findings that the opportunity to perform new

TABLE 3. Transfer of Training Regression Model

	Beta	Standard Error	Standard Beta	t	Sig.
Constant	16.90	8.62	----	1.96	.05
Learning Outcomes (Time 1)	.60	.08	.53	8.01	.00
Opportunity to Perform	1.75	.47	.26	3.75	.00
Post-Training Peer Support	1.23	.58	.14	2.12	.04
Familiarity with Content	−2.63	1.06	−.16	−2.48	.02

R = .74, Adjusted R Square = .52, Standard Error of the Estimate = 13.21

tasks and post-training peer support were predictors of participant's evaluation of attaining the learning outcomes is consistent with the literature.

DISCUSSION AND RECOMMENDATIONS

The evaluation approach presented here used a transfer of training model that included asking trainees to provide their perceptions of how well they attained the specified learning outcomes at the end of training as well as six months later. They also reported their perceptions of personal and organizational factors that the literature suggests are important to the transfer of new learning to the job.

There are several limitations to this study. The transfer literature is just beginning to identify the variables that might explain the use of new skills after training. At this point of development there is no widely accepted model of transfer that can be tested. Similarly, there are no standardized measures of the variables that are identified in the literature. This study used some measures from previous studies, developed others, and pilot tested the instruments. The validity and reliability of the instruments has not been firmly established, however.

The dependent variable in this study was worker self-report of the attainment of learning outcomes as measured by the change in their assessment over time. Clearly, a better measure of what was learned in training and used on the job is needed in future research. A combination of self-report and supervisor report would be a stronger measure. If sufficient resources were available, behavioral assessment pre-training, immediately post-training and six months later would be better.

In addition, this was a survey where the follow-up questionnaire was sent by mail. While the response rate for this survey of 51% is acceptable, the results for those not responding could greatly change the study findings. Even with the limitations of this study, the findings are useful for continued research in this field as well as for consideration in designing training. Every aspect of the transfer of training to the job is deserving of further research.

One important implication for training design that comes from this study was the negative relationship between participant's report of obtaining the learning outcomes and their familiarity with the content. On average trainees reported that they knew 60% of the material prior to attending training. This variable is part of what is identified in the literature as decision involvement. One method for addressing both trainee decision involvement and the work-related relevance of the training is through self-assessment of training needs (Baldwin & Ford, 1988; Curry et al., 1994; Ford & Noe, 1987; Guthrie &

Schwoerer, 1994). Ideally supervisors and workers would engage in a guided skill assessment process on a periodic basis. From this assessment both parties could develop a plan for skill development that would identify training that both believe to be beneficial. An employee self-assessment completed prior to training would also allow employees the opportunity to determine their own training needs and promotes a sense of investment in the training process (Baldwin & Ford, 1988; Ford & Noe, 1987, Pecora, 1989). Results of this study suggest that greater involvement by trainees in the training process may positively influence their learning of new skills and their ability to transfer them to the job. When joint or self-assessments are not feasible due to concerns about accuracy and work setting characteristics, the options of using job performance evaluations, focus groups, and/or agency outcomes to determine training needs remain viable (Denning & Verschelden, 1993; Pecora et al., 1983). No matter what method is used to assess training needs, the perception of training utility and the level of trainee involvement are key in influencing conditions that contribute to transfer of training (Ford & Noe, 1987).

Opportunity to perform new learning after completion of training and peer support for applying new learning were found to be important factors explaining training transfer. Higher levels of opportunity to perform and peer support were associated with greater learning and application of new skills. The two elements of opportunity to perform are supervisors providing workers both with tasks that allow the use of new skills and the time to practice and implement new skills. Elements of peer support include being able to talk with colleagues about the training experience and the support of peers in attempting to use new skills.

The supervisor is key to structuring opportunities to practice new skills as well as creating a work climate that promotes peer support for applying new learning. One strategy for doing this is for the supervisor to confer with caseworkers about how to integrate what they have learned in training with current cases and job responsibilities. They can also establish expectations for their team to try new learning and support each other for these attempts.

There were some secondary findings that are worthy of consideration. Based on trainee feedback, the setting of post-training goals was not encouraged during the course of training. The transfer literature advises that an effort should be made to include goal setting into the training experience. Trainers are well positioned to assist trainees in setting such goals. Post-training plans could also be developed during the course of training. Trainers might even find a feasible way of following up with participants after they have returned to the field.

There were other factors identified in the literature as important to training transfer that were not included in the final model. It is interesting that supervisor support prior to training was not a significant predictor of learning outcomes. Because of the important role that supervisors play in the pre-training environment one wonders if the results would have been different if there had been more pre-training supervisory support. The literature suggests that it is important for supervisors to reflect a positive attitude regarding the workers opportunity to attend training and to encourage them to share what they learn upon their return. In addition, another key supervisory activity that may contribute to a positive pre-training environment is to assist in making plans for the worker caseloads to be covered during the training period. The supervisor may also be the key to influencing the level of peer support that staff receives prior to attending a training event since supervisors who value training are likely to have staff members share similar perceptions and provide support for one another.

The individual attributes of training participants that are identified in the literature as important to training transfer did not appear in the model that resulted in this study. Self-efficacy, for example, was significant at the bivariate level but did not enter the model. While not significant in this study it is worth considering that providing performance feedback to trainees is a viable way to shape and encourage their feelings of self-efficacy (Karl et al., 1993).

CONCLUSION

The study reported here represents a useful step toward the development of a tool designed to be responsive to a critical question: *Is the amount of time and money spent on child welfare training achieving the intended results in the field?* The results of this exploratory study helped to identify variables that are key to influencing the transfer of training and also suggest viable steps that agencies committed to maximizing the benefits of training for child welfare practice can take to increase the return on their investment. A foundation has also been laid for continuing research efforts aimed at developing and refining an evaluative tool that addresses the transfer of training issue.

NOTE

1. All scales used in this study are available from the authors. The item responses for the scales ranged from strongly disagree (1) to strongly agree (6).

REFERENCES

Baldwin, T. T., & Ford, J. K. (1988). Transfer of training: A review and directions for future research. *Personnel Psychology, 41,* 63-101.
Bandura, A. (1986). *Social foundations of thought and action: A social cognitive theory.* Englewood Cliffs, New Jersey: Prentice Hall.

Bennett, J. B., Lehman, Wayne, E. K., & Forst, J. K. (1999). Change, transfer climate, and customer orientation: A contextual model and analysis of change driven training. *Group & Organization Management 24* (2), 188-216.

Bowne, A. W. (1999). The field study of a training transfer enhancement process and its effect on transfer of training. *Dissertation Abstracts International, 60* (3-1).

Clark, C. S. (1991). Social processes in work groups: A model of the effect of involvement, credibility, and goal linkage on training success. *Dissertation Abstracts International, 52* (3-A).

Clark, C., Dobbins, G., & Ladd, R. (1993). Exploratory field study of training motivation. *Group & Organization Management, 18* (3), 292-307.

Curry, D. H., Caplan, P., & Knuppel, J. (1994). Transfer of training and adult learning (TOTAL). *Journal of Continuing Social Work Education, 6* (1), 8-14.

Denning, J. D. & Verschelden, C. (1993). Using the focus group in assessing training needs: Empowering child welfare workers. *Child Welfare, 72* (6), 569-79.

Dottalo, P. (1994). A comparison of discriminant analysis and logistic progression. *Journal of Social Service Research, 19*, pp. 121-144.

Doucek, H. J. & Austin, M. J. (1986). Improving agency functioning through staff development. *Administration in Social Work, 10* (2), 27-37.

Erera, I. P. & Lazar, A. (1993). Training needs of social work supervisors. *Clinical Supervisor, 11* (1), 83-93.

Ford, J. K. & Noe, R. A. (1987). Self-assessed training needs: The effects of attitudes toward training, managerial level, and function. *Personnel Psychology, 40,* 39-53.

Ford, J. K., Quinones, M. A., Sego, D. J., & Sorra, J. S. (1992). Factors affecting the opportunity to perform trained tasks on the job. *Personnel Psychology, 45,* 511-526.

Garavaglia, P. L. (1993). How to ensure transfer of training. *Training and Development, 47,* 63-68.

Gregoire, T. K. (1994). Assessing the benefits and increasing the utility of addiction training for public child welfare workers: A pilot study. *Child Welfare, 73,* 69-81.

Gregoire, T. K., Propp, J., & Poertner, J. (1998). The supervisor's role in transfer of training. *Administration in Social Work, vol. 22,* (1), 1-18.

Guthrie, J. P., & Schwoerer, C. E. (1994). Individual and contextual influences on self-assessed training needs. *Journal of Organizational Behavior, 15*, 405-422.

Hagan, J. (1990). Training income maintenance workers: A look at the empirical evidence. *Journal of Continuing Social Work Education, 5* (2), 3-8.

Karl, K. A., O'Leary-Kelly, A. M., & Martocchio, J. J. (1993). The impact of feedback and self-efficacy on performance in training. *Journal of Organizational Behavior, 14,* 379-394.

Kozlowski, S. W., & Doherty, M. L. (1989). Integration of climate and leadership: Examination of a neglected issue. *Journal of Applied Psychology, 74* (4), 546-553.

Latham, G. P. (1988). Human resource training and development. *Annual Review of Psychology, 39*, 545-582.

McDonald, R. M. (1991). Assessment of organizational context: A missing component in evaluations of training programs. *Evaluation and Program Planning,* 14, 273-279.

Miller, J. & Dore, M. M. (1991). Innovations in child protective services inservice training: Commitment to excellence. *Child Welfare, 65* (4), 437-449.

Morin, L. (1999). Mental practice and goal-setting as transfer of training strategies: Their influence on self-efficacy and task performance of team leaders in an organizational setting. *Dissertation Abstracts International 60* (1-A).

Noe, R. A. (1986). Trainee's attributes and attitudes: Neglected influences on training effectiveness. *Academy of Management Review, 11* (4), 736-749.

Noe, R. A. & Schmitt, N. (1986). The influence of trainer attitudes on training effectiveness: Test of a model. *Personnel Psychology, 39,* 497-523.

Olivero, G., Bane, K. D., & Kopelman, R. E. (1997). Executive coaching as a transfer of training tool: Effects on productivity in a public agency. *Public Personnel Management, 26* (4) 461-469.

Pecora, P. J. (1989). Improving the quality of child welfare services: Needs assessment for staff training. *Child Welfare, 68* (4), 403-418.

Pecora, P. J., Dodson, A. R., Teather, E. C., & Whittaker, J. K. (1983). Assessing worker training needs: Use of staff surveys and key informant interviews. *Child Welfare, 62* (5), 395-407.

Rooney, R. H. (1988). Measuring task-centered training effects on practice: Results of an audiotape study in a public agency. *Journal of Continuing Social Work Education, 4* (4), 2-7.

Seipel, M. M. (1986). Staff training policies in public child welfare agencies: A quest for rationality. *Journal of Continuing Social Work Education, 4* (1), 25-29.

Tannenbaum, S. I. & Yukl, G. (1992). Training and development in work organizations. *Annual Review of Psychology, 43,* 399-441.

Tziner, A., Haccoun, R. R., & Kadish, A. (1991). Personal and situational characteristics influencing the effectiveness of transfer of training improvement strategies. *Journal of Occupational Psychology, 64,* 167-177.

U.S. Department of Health and Human Services Administration for Children and Families. (2000). "Protecting the well-being of children" [Online]. Available: www.acf.dhhs.gov/programs/opa/facts/chilwel.htm.

U.S. Government Printing Office. (1998). Section 11. Child protection, foster care, and adoption. *1998 Green Book* [Online]. Available: http://frwebgate./access.gpo.gov.

Vinokur-Kaplan, D. (1987). A national survey of in-service training experiences of child welfare supervisors and worker. *Social Service Review,* pp. 291-304.

Wright, W. S., & Fraser, M. (1988). Staff development: A challenge of privatization. *Journal of Continuing Social Work Education, 4*(4), 137-159.

A Follow-Up of a Title IV-E Program's Graduates' Retention Rates in a Public Child Welfare Agency

Loring Jones, DSW

SUMMARY. *Objective*: Examine retention rates of a Title IV-E program's graduates in a public child welfare agency. *Method:* The sample consisted of all workers (N = 266) hired between June 1994 and June 1997. Subjects were followed until 12/31/99 in order to ascertain employment status. Data for study were abstracted from agency personnel files. *Findings:* Title IV-E trained social workers had longer periods of tenure than non-IV-E trained employees (p < .057). Other predictors that were significant or approaching significance included Spanish speaking (p < .007), having an MSW (p < .0245), being rehired by the agency (p < .052), and being promoted to social from Income Maintenance (p < .061). *Conclusions:* The retention finding is encouraging because it may mean child welfare agencies may improve their human capital through programs like IV-E. Recruiting Spanish speaking social workers or upgrading existing workers' language skills may increase retention in child welfare. Promoting from within coupled with upgrading skills through training programs like IV-E may also be a solution to the staffing crisis. *[Article copies available for a fee from The Haworth Document Delivery Service: 1-800-HAWORTH. E-mail address: <getinfo@haworthpressinc.com> Website: <http://www.HaworthPress.com> © 2002 by The Haworth Press, Inc. All rights reserved.]*

Loring Jones is Professor of Social Work, San Diego State University.

[Haworth co-indexing entry note]: "A Follow-Up of a Title IV-E Program's Graduates' Retention Rates in a Public Child Welfare Agency." Jones, Loring. Co-published simultaneously in *Journal of Health & Social Policy* (The Haworth Press, Inc.) Vol. 15, No. 3/4, 2002, pp. 39-51; and: *Evaluation Research in Child Welfare: Improving Outcomes Through University-Public Agency Partnerships* (ed: Katharine Briar-Lawson, and Joan Levy Zlotnik) The Haworth Press, Inc., 2002, pp. 39-51. Single or multiple copies of this article are available for a fee from The Haworth Document Delivery Service [1-800-HAWORTH, 9:00 a.m. - 5:00 p.m. (EST). E-mail address: getinfo@haworthpressinc.com].

KEYWORDS. Retention, turnover, child welfare, Title IV-E

INTRODUCTION

Recruiting and retaining social workers for child welfare practice has been a concern for some time (Pecora, Briar, and Zlotnick, 1989). Retaining recruited workers is a cause for concern because it negatively affects health and human services agencies in a number of ways. First, agencies must compete with one another for a limited number of candidates. Many social workers do not wish to work in public child welfare, and the loss of a worker diminishes that pool even further. Second, the replacement cost per worker (estimated to be between $15,000 and $17,000), turnover can be a substantial strain on an agency's budget (Daly, Dudley, Finnegan Jones, and Christiansen, 2000). This estimate includes costs associated with advertisement, recruitment, orientation, induction training, and time devoted to reduced caseload during training. Turnover often causes employee morale to diminish, resulting in even higher level of employee turnover. Finally, and perhaps most seriously, failure to retain employees represents a loss of human capital (i.e., the cost of replacing experienced workers with inexperienced workers).

This paper examines retention among Title IV-E graduates in one Southern California public child welfare agency. The Title IV-E training program was developed by the California Social Work Education (CALSWEC) to reprofessionalize child welfare practice. The Title IV-E training program is based on the assumption that social workers can provide more effective child welfare services than staff who do not have professional social work training. Considerable resources were expended by the California schools to develop social workers who have the skills and competencies to work in child welfare. There has always been some anxiety by CALSWEC designers about whether the IV-E workers would choose to remain in public child welfare practice once there employment obligations were completed. This paper is part of an ongoing project to examine graduates employment history in child welfare, and to compare their turnover and retention rates in child welfare.

LITERATURE REVIEW

In order for public child welfare agencies to carry out their mission, they must have quality, well-educated, and trained staffs (Terpestra, 1992; Siu and Hogan, 1988). A number of researchers have provided some documentation that professional social work provides the necessary knowledge and skills for practice in public social service (Booz-Allen, 1987; Lieberman, Hornby, and Russell, 1988; Pecora, Briar, and Zlotnik, 1989). However, public child welfare agencies often encounter problems attracting and retaining social workers stemming from large caseloads, diminishing resources, unclear practice and policy guidelines, controversial public images of the agency and worker, perceptions of child welfare as a low status career, lack of career ladders, low pay, insufficient training opportunities, inadequate supervision, excessive bureaucracy, and stressful work environments (Kahn and Kamerman, 1989; Pecora, Briar, and Zlotnik, 1989; Russel, 1987, Rycraft, 1994, and Vinokur-Kaplan and Hartman, 1986). Also contributing to the decline of employment in public sectors was the disappearance of funding for child welfare training stipends caused by the block granting of Title XX funds (Harris, 1992). In addition, the declassification of public child welfare positions during the 1980s, prompted in part by the lack of social workers applying for public sectors jobs, resulted in the lowering of educational requirements for these positions (Millar and Dore, 1991; National Center for Social Policy and Practice, 1989).

These changes diminished the incentives for professional social workers to practice in public child welfare. Agencies increasingly hired individuals without formal training in social work (Russel, 1988). A study assessing the educational background of 5,000 personnel found that only 28% had a degree in social work. Three-quarters of these personnel had only BA degrees. Most of the BA level practitioners had degrees in fields other than social work. Only fifteen percent of the personnel had bachelor's degrees in social work (Lieberman, Hornby, and Russel, 1988). The shortfall in the number of professionally trained public child welfare professionals is drastic. A survey conducted by the California Chapter of NASW in 1987-88 found that only 23% of child welfare workers had an MSW degree, and one-third of the counties in California do not have any masters level social workers employed in child welfare services (Laughlin and Specht, 1992). Estimates drawn from a national survey conducted by the Child Welfare League of America (CWLA, 1990) found that child welfare practitioners in public agencies had lower educational levels than workers in private agencies.

Public child welfare programs have been subject to intense public scrutiny in recent years, often in connection with deaths or injuries of children in placement, or with disruption of families that might have been preserved. These incidents often reflect the pressure of caseloads that are rapidly increasing in numbers and severity while resources are diminished. Often, however, workers who have committed serious practice errors have been poorly trained in the legal requirements and complex skills associated with child welfare practice. In several states, child protective services agencies have been found by the courts to be deficient in observing legal and professional practice standards. Consent decrees agreed to by states and counties have included requirements for upgrading child welfare staff. These decrees indicate hiring preferences for persons with human services or social work degrees (Stein, 1991).

Historically, social work has been the predominant profession in child welfare. Several studies have shown the relevance of social work training for child welfare practice (Booz-Allen, 1987). However, the social work literature describes a widespread abandonment in the last two decades of child welfare by social work (Costin, Bell, and Downs, 1991; Jaratatne and Chess, 1983; Lieberman, Hornby, and Russel, 1988; Grossman, Laughlin, and Specht, 1992; Harris, 1992). Many social work educators and their students view public agency practice as undesirable, while many public agency managers view social work curriculums as irrelevant. Increasingly social workers are leaving or avoiding public child welfare (Harrison, 1980; Pecora, Whittaker and Maluccio, 1992).

Vulnerable children and families are often ill-served by the public child welfare system. These children and families must contend with agencies that are understaffed, overburdened, and deficient in resources to meet human need. The lack of professional social workers employed in child welfare renders these agencies unable to meet the legislative mandates and professional standards required for employees working in child welfare.

The California IV-E MSW Child Welfare Program was created in 1991 in response to the drastic shortage of MSW staff in California child welfare divisions (less than 30%), and the dramatic increase in reports of child maltreatment (119,000 in 1976 to 555,782 in 1990) (Clark and Grossman, 1992).

CALSWEC is a joint effort of the fourteen California graduate schools of social welfare, the fifty-eight county welfare directors, the National Association of Social Workers, mental health representatives, and private foundations. The mission of CALSWEC is to reprofessionalize public social services particularly in child welfare and mental health. The California Department of Social Services entered into a contract in 1992 with the CALSWEC to increase the number of MSW's practicing in California public child welfare services. Grant funds were secured through Title IV-E of the Social Security Act in January 1993.

PROGRAM DESCRIPTION

The School of Social Work at San Diego State University (SDSU-SSW) has been a key participant in the development of CALSWEC at the local level. SDSU-SSW initiated a collaborative process with the San Diego County Department of Social Services, Childrens Services Bureau (DSS) to meet CALSWEC's goals.

Full-time MSW students admitted to the School of Social Work are eligible to apply for the Title IV-E stipend of $18,000 per academic year. The stipend amount for IV-E workers reported upon in this paper was $15,000. A group of additional students employed at DSS receive educational reimbursement funds to attend the IV-E program part-time. Applicants are selected by a joint stipend awards committee made up of equal number of representatives from the county agencies and the school faculty. Priority is given to Department of Social Services employees and to students who have the capacity and commitment to serve a diverse population in public child welfare. The intent of CALSWEC is to seek students who consider child welfare a career track, and would be committed to a career in child welfare (Fong, 1994). Students sign agreements which require payback of the stipend through post-MSW employment in a child protective services position in any county agency within the State of California, or if they are an American Indian with tribal registration, in an Indian serving agency. For every year of stipend, the graduate must payback a calendar year of employment which also applies to employed students receiving reimbursements. For most students the payback period is two years. Title IV-E funded students must also agree to abide by the requirements of the child welfare practice curriculum set by each school based on the CALSWEC child welfare competencies, including at least one year of field internship in the public child welfare agency. Each year 20 full-time MSW students enter the program. One hundred twenty-five MSWs have completed the child welfare curriculum under the Title IV-E stipend program at San Diego State University.

The SDSU curriculum for Children, Youth, and Families was redesigned to match the knowledge and skill acquisitions objectives of CALSWEC. The SDSU Title IV-E program is formulated on the premise that specific child welfare competency based training will lead to a competent practitioner, who will more likely make child welfare a career, than workers without that training. These practitioners will more likely be able to deal with the demands and stresses of child protective service practice, and are more likely to remain employed than workers without such training. As such the IV-E program is an attempt to reprofessionalize child welfare practice.

METHODOLOGY

This study is a follow-up of an earlier study (Jones and Okamura, 2000). The initial study followed new hires in Children Services of the Department of Social Services (DSS) from June 1994 until June 1997 in order to obtain employment status information. Retention and termination rates were examined and compared for IV-E trained workers and non-IV-E trained workers. The current study updates employment status of those workers through December 31, 1999. All IV-E workers had completed the required payback by June of 1999. In the first study only 50% of the graduates had completed payback.

Sample

This sample represents all new hires to the Children's Services Bureau between June of 1994 and August of 1996. Thirty-five transfers from the Income Maintenance Bureau of DSS were part of the sample since they were new to the Children's Services Bureau, and attended initial training. DSS–San Diego is made up of two parts, The Children's Service Bureau (CSB), which provides child protective services, and the Income Maintenance Bureau, which administers public assistance programs. Workers can transfer between Bureaus as they obtain seniority and positions become vacant. Thirty-nine workers in the sample were IV-E trained. Two-hundred-twenty-seven non-IV-E new hires served as a comparison group.

The IV-E workers had graduated SDSU in either 1994 or 1995.Thirty-three other IV-E graduates who returned to positions at DSS after graduate school are not part of the evaluation. They were excluded from the study because it was assumed that their status as long time DSS employees might confound a retention study that included new hires. Four other IV-E graduates were excluded because they took positions in other parts of California. The entire sample went through a five week initial training program at DSS prior to being assigned a caseload. The initial training included content on basic practice, policy, and procedures unique to the agency. Practice training was based on the Institute of Human Services–Child Welfare League of America competencies (Institute for Human Services, 1992).

Data Collection

All 266 employees hired between the Summer or 1994 and 1995 were followed until the December 31, 1999 in order to ascertain their employment status. The study was a retrospective descriptive case record analysis. The specific aim of the research was to determine if there were differences in retention rates between IV-E trained students and other workers.

Two study groups are available for comparisons on outcomes. The first group is made up IV-E workers and the other of non-IV-E workers.

Study data were derived from case record review of employees personnel records. Data in these files describes the employment history in the agency and some demographic characteristics. An instrument was developed to abstract data from the case files. Collection of data was carried out by a social work graduate research assistant who was trained by a member of the DSS personnel office to abstract relevant data from the file.

FINDINGS

Tables 1 and 2 provide a description of the sample at the time they were hired by the agency. Chi-square was used with nominal level data and t-tests were used with interval level data.

Demographic and professional variables are assumed to affect how long a person is able to stay on the job. Title IV-E graduates were younger and were less likely to have children than the comparisons. IV-E respondents were more

TABLE 1. Description of the Sample–Demographics

Variable	IV-E Graduates (N = 39)	Non-IV-E Workers (N = 227)	
Average Age in Years	31.6 (sd = 8.98)	36.0 (sd = 9.95)	p < .009
% married & living w/ spouse	48.3	46.8	
% divorced	0	15.1	
% single	37.9	27.8	
% separated	3.4	1.6	
% domestic partnership	10.3	8.7	
% with children	19.2	50.0	p < .001
% White	44.4	66.3	p < .03
% Black	13.9	8.7	
% Hispanic	23.1	19.2	
% Asian	16.7	2.3	
% Spanish speaking*	15.4	12.8	
% male	9	17.1	p < .01

*DSS provides bilingual pay of 10% increment in pay for Spanish speaking workers. They are also supposed to receive a 10% caseload reduction in exchange for providing translation services for other workers. Most Spanish speaking workers report they do not receive this reduction, but that they still provide translation services. Other bilingual speakers do not receive this pay. The rationale for only providing Spanish speakers with this pay is that about 23% of children receiving services from DSS come from Hispanic families. Other language groups are only a fraction of that percentage.

TABLE 2. Description of the Sample–Professional Experience Percentage and Means Reported

Variable	IV-E Graduates (N = 39)	Non-IV-E Workers (N = 168)
% with MSWs (total = 48%)	100%	26.9 %
% with MA degrees	100%	52.4%
# of yrs worked in soc. serv.	3.6	5.5 (P < .05)
# of yrs worked with children	2.6	3.8 (P < .15)
% who were eligibility workers	17.1 %	13.9 %
Spanish speaking*	15%	12 %

*fluent Spanish speakers receive a pay premium

likely to be female and minority group members than the non-IV-E trained comparisons. IV-E recruiting policies gives preferences to minorities.

The sample had a great deal of human capital. Seventy-seven percent of the sample (N = 266) had a master's degree. Forty-eight percent had an MSW. Most of the MSWs in the sample had attended SDSU, but only IV-E graduates had the educational program described earlier in this paper. The remainder of the master's degrees were mostly Marriage and Family Counselors (MFCC). Psychologists and counselors can have the MFCC certification. Twenty-one workers (8%) went through an MFCC program. Non-IV-E workers had more practice experience, including experience working with children than the IV-E respondents. The BA workers were mostly former eligibility workers and Spanish speaking workers. A small number of long time employees had BA degrees and had been "grandfathered" into positions before the agency expressed a preference for graduate level workers The eligibility workers were able to obtain their position without a masters because of an agency promote from within policy. At the current time the only BA level workers hired from outside the agency are fluent Spanish speakers. A large portion of the agency caseload is made up of Spanish speaking families, and master's level Spanish speakers are in short supply. MSWs and Spanish speakers receive a small salary differential of about 5% of their salary. Title IV-E workers receive the MSW increment, but they receive no extra pay for their graduate child welfare training.

Table 3 reports the employment status of the sample on 12/30/99 approximately 4 1/2 years after data collection began. Table 4 reports the sample's length of employment in days. Each variable in Table 3 and 4 is dichotomous. Significance was determined by the chi-square.

TABLE 3. Percentage Still Employed at DSS as of December 31, 1999 (Dependent Variable)

Independent Variables	Percentage Still Employed	Significance
Title IV-E (N = 39)	69.2	p < .165
MSW (N = 100)	65.0	NS
Non-IV-E MSWs (N = 61)	62.3	NS
Master's Level (N = 208)	58.7	NS
Non-MSW Master's (N = 59)	64.3	NS
Spanish Speaking (N = 39)	82.1	p < .007
BA or less Level (N = 50)	57.1	NS
Eligibility Worker (N = 35)	74.3	p < .061
Male (N = 67)	59.7	NS
Female (N = 199)	61.3	NS
African American (N = 21)	66.7	NS
Hispanic (N = 52)	69.2	NS
White (N = 133)*	68.1	NS
Overall (N = 266)	59.6	

*Asians and American Indians not reported because of small N. Also difference from 100% is a result of missing data.

One hundred and four workers (39.1%) had left DSS during the period of observation. Thirty percent of the IV-E workers had left during the period (p < .165). The mean length of employment for the sample was 1118.92 days. The IV-E workers remained employed at DSS for an average of 12995.56 days (p < .057). Non-IV-E trained MSWs did not have a significantly longer period of tenure than either other master's level workers or the BA level workers. However, MSWs had longer period of employment as measured in number of days of employment than non-MSWs (p < .024). Rehires were more likely to be continued employment than other workers.

Spanish speakers were more likely to remain at DSS than other workers. Surprisingly, this relationship does not hold true for Hispanic workers in general. Most, eighty-two percent, of the bilingual workers were Hispanic. Workers promoted from the Income Maintenance Bureau were also more likely to have remained employed, but the difference is only approaching significance (p > .065). Younger workers were also more likely to leave (p < .024). None of the demographic variables predicted either exit or length of tenure.

TABLE 4. Length of Employment at DSS in Days (Dependent Variable) (n = 266)

Independent Variables	Number of Days	Significance
Title IV-E	1295.56 (sd = 562.83)	p < .057
MSW	1229.63 (sd = 639.74)	p < .024
Non-IV-E MSWs	1174.91 (sd = 692.42)	NS
Master's Level	1168.85 (sd = 633.49)	p < .104
Bilingual	1275.77 (sd = 572.64)	p < .10
BA Level or Less	1029.5 (sd = 648.48)	p < .094
Eligibility Worker	1228.03 (sd = 459.93)	p < .10
Male	1061.38 (sd = 598.98)	NS
Female	1138.49 (sd = 661.18)	NS
African American	1187.43 (sd = 754.97)	NS
Hispanic	1056.83 (sd = 586.36)	NS
Rehire	1572.54 (sd = 773.6)	p < .0001
Non-MSW MAs	1135.69 (sd = 615.78)	NS
Overall	1118.92 (sd = 645.72)	—-

CONCLUSIONS

Title IV-E workers were more likely to have remained employed for a longer period of time than non-IV-E workers. However, this finding was only at a level that indicates a trend. Only bilingual status predicted at a significant level whether one was employed or not. Trending toward significance in predicting employment in addition to IV-E status was having an MSW or other masters, having transferred from eligibility, and having been rehired by the agency. The rehire variable and having an MSW were the only variables that significantly predicted the number of days employed. IV-E status, bilingual authorization, having a master's degree, having been an eligibility worker also were also trending toward predicting length of days employed.

The IV-E finding suggests that dedicated and experienced cadre might choose to remain in public child welfare over the long term. This finding needs investigation because it is only approaching significance, but is encouraging because it may mean that the long standing staffing crisis in child welfare may have a solution in programs like IV-E. If the staffing crisis is resolved it is possible to improve practice in an overburdened child welfare system. The MSW findings may also suggest more of a willingness of MSWs in general to practice in child welfare.

IV-E workers entered the agency with a more realistic view of IV-E practice than most of the new hires. This realistic view may have helped workers adapt to DSS practice. These workers may not stay unless the unsatisfactory working conditions identified in the literature of this paper are changed. Schools must realize that only one half of the job is to train workers. The second half of the task is to work with agency administrators to help them develop working conditions that are conducive to workers remaining in the agency. Otherwise, in the long run, these programs may fail as workers exit the agency to find more satisfactory working environments.

Applicants for employment at DSS might be warned about potential sources of job dissatisfaction and stress. A dose of realism during interviews and initial training might reduce cost of expensive short-term periods of employment. Beginning initial training with field observations, and presentations from panels of veteran workers might provide that realism. Initial training and ongoing should provide workshops on how to manage to stress. On-going in-service training in stress management may be another strategy to help retain workers. Workers should learn self-care strategies, the pitfalls of over involvement, the limits of services, how to leave the job at work, and about the difficulties of how to manage personal feelings in a difficult job are all something workers need to know. Supervisors should have training in identifying and intervening when their workers are in crisis.

Data also suggests that Spanish speaking workers were more likely to stay. About a quarter of the agencies caseload is made up of Spanish speaking families. Spanish speaking workers receive a salary increment for their language skills. Salary increments might encourage workers to remain on the job. They may also derive a sense of accomplishment from their use of language skills. Many of these workers were BA level workers, but their fellow master's level workers often relied on them to translate for Spanish speaking clients. They may also recognize their linguistic and cultural skills contributed much to the families in their caseload. Teaching Spanish to MSWs preparing for a career in child welfare may be a way of contributing to longer stays in the public child welfare program.

Eligibility workers were also slightly more likely to remain at DSS. These workers may have learned some skills in income maintenance to help them do their jobs in child protection. They also may have developed a commitment to the agency from their previous employment, and have accrued vacation and retirements benefits that made continued employment attractive. Most of these workers were BA level workers. Balfour and Neff (1993), in a study of retention in child welfare, found caseworkers that were most likely to stay were those with a bachelor's degree and at least two years of service with the agency preceded by relevant internship experience. Additionally, caseworkers working for agencies with few pay differentials and advancement opportunities were less likely to leave than were new workers (i.e., caseworker with less than two years employment with the agency) with no previous experience in human services. The probability of leaving increased for those with master's degrees and limited overtime hours. Thus, the authors suggest that one way to reduce turnover is to focus on staff with more education, less experience, and less stake in the organization. A lesson of the current study is that one way to fight high turnover is to promote from within and use IV-E programs to have workers upgrade their skills.

Rehires were most likely to stay. Perhaps after seeing other field of service they decided that CPS employment was not that difficult. Agencies are often reluctant to re-hire workers who have left, but these data suggest they may represent a dedicated group of workers if they can be encouraged to return. Sabbaticals for workers in agencies which would allow them to get away and recharge their energies might lead to more workers with long-term employment.

This evaluation only examined employment variables. Evaluating the effectiveness of the IV-E program should also consist of an examination of how workers actually perform the job. Some outcomes that could be investigated include: Do MSWs in public child welfare carry a larger volume of difficult cases? Do their caseloads contain more difficult cases? Do IV-E trained workers accomplish case goals more quickly than their counterparts. IV-E training program is based on the assumption that social workers can provide more effective child welfare services than staff who do not have this training. This assumption needs to be tested.

REFERENCES

Balfour, D. and Neff, D. (1993). Predicting and managing turnover in human service agencies: A case study of an organization in crisis. *Public Personnel Management,* 22 (3), 473-486.

Booz-Allen and Hamilton, Inc. (January, 1987). *The Maryland Social Work Services Job Analysis and Personal Qualifications Study.* Silver Spring, MD: NASW.

Clark, S. and Grossman, B. (April, 1992). The California Competency-Based Child Welfare Curriculum Project. Report of the Curriculum Sub-Committee. Berkeley: University of California, California Social Work Education Center.

Costin, L., Bell, C., and Downs, S. (1991). *Child Welfare Practices and Policies.* New York: Longman Publishing.

CWLA. (1990). Salary Study–1989. Washington, DC: Child Welfare League of America.

Daly, D, Dudley, D., Finnegan, D., and Christiansen (2000). Staffing Child Welfare Services in the New Millennium. San Diego, CA: Network for Excellence.

Fong, T. (1994). Child Welfare Field Instructor Resource Manual. California IV-E MSW Child Welfare Program. San Diego: SDSU School of Social Work..

Grossman, B., Laughlin, S., and Specht, H. (1992). *Building Commitment of Social Work Education to Publically Supported Social Services: The California Model.* In the proceeding from "New Partnerships." The National Public Child Welfare Training Symposium. Florida International University, Miami, FL.

Harris, N. (1992). *Social Work Education and Public Human Services Partnerships: A Technical Assistance Document.* A report of a Ford Foundation funded project and the Council on Social Work Education.

Harrison, W. D. (1980). Role strain and burnout in child protective service workers. *Social Service Review, 54,* 31-44.

Institute for Human Services. (1992). Competencies for a Master's Level Educational Specialization in Child Welfare Practice. Columbus, OH: Institute for Human Services.

Jayraratne, S., Vinokur-Caplan, D., and Chess, W. (1993). The importance of personal control: A comparison of private practice and public agency settings. Unpublished paper. School of Social Work, University of Michigan.

Jones, L. and Okamura, A. (2000). Reprofessionalizing Child Welfare Services: An evaluation of a Title IV-E Training Program. *Research on Social Work Practice,* Vol. 22, (5), pp. 355-371.

Kahn, A. and Kammerman, S. (1989). *Social Services in the United States.* Philadelphia: Temple University Press, 485-492.

Lieberman, A., Hornby, H., and Russel, M. (1988). Analyzing the educational backgrounds and work experience of child welfare personnel: A national study. *Social Work, 33,* 485-492.

Millar, K. (1986). Declassification of professional social workers: A personnel issue facing human services. *Administration in Social Work, 10,* 15-20.

Miller, J. and Dore, M. (1991). Innovations in child protective service inservice training. *Child Welfare, 60,* 437-449.

National Center for Social Policy and Practice. (1989). *Social Workers in Public Social Services: A Review of the Literature.* Silver Spring, MD: NASW.

Pecora, P., Briar, K., and Zlotnick, J. (1989). *Addressing the Program and Personnel Crisis in Child Welfare.* Silver Spring, MD: NASW.

Pecora, P., Whittaker, J., and Maluccio. (1992). The child welfare challenge: Policy, practice, and research. New York: Walter de Gruyter.

Russel, M. (1988). *Public Child Welfare Job Requirements.* Portland, ME: National Child Welfare Resource Center for Management and Administration.

Rycraft. (1994). The party isn't over: The agency role in the retention of public child welfare workers. *Social Work,* 39, 75-80.

Siu, S. and Hogan, P. (1989). Public child welfare: The need for clinical social work. *Social Work, 34,* 385-400.

Stein, T. (1991). *Child Welfare and the Law.* New York: Longman Publishing.

Terpestra, J. (1992). *Forward to New Partnerships.* In the proceeding from "New Partnerships" The National Public Child Welfare Training Symposium. Florida International University, Miami, FL.

Tracy, E., Bean, N., Gwatkin, S., and Hill, B. (1994). Family preservation workers: Sources of job satisfaction and job stress. *Research on Social Work Practice,* 2, 465-478.

Vinokur-Kaplan, D. and Hartman, A. (1986). A national profile of child welfare workers and supervisors. *Child Welfare, 65,* 323-335.

Career Paths and Contributions of Four Cohorts of IV-E Funded MSW Child Welfare Graduates

Sandra C. Robin, PhD
C. David Hollister, PhD

SUMMARY. For the last decade the federal government has provided financial support through Title IV-E of the Social Security Act to schools of social work to provide professional education in child welfare. This study looks at the first four cohorts of graduates who received IV-E funding from one school of social work. Data on MSW graduates from 1993-1996 (N = 73), as well as survey responses (N = 32), were analyzed to ascertain dimensions of their career development in, and contributions to, child welfare social work. Results indicate that the vast majority of graduates funded by IV-E dollars became employed in and stayed in child welfare focused social work, with a strong percentage in public child welfare services, and that these social work-educated social workers are actively involved in shaping the practice, policies and administration of child welfare services. *[Article copies available for a fee from The Haworth Document Delivery Service: 1-800-HAWORTH. E-mail address:*

Sandra C. Robin is Associate Professor in the Department of Social Work, St. Cloud State University, St. Cloud, MN. At the time of this research she was Associate Director of the Center for Advanced Studies in Child Welfare, School of Social Work, University of Minnesota, St. Paul, MN.

C. David Hollister is Professor in the School of Social Work, University of Minnesota, St. Paul, MN, and is Program Evaluator of the Center for Advanced Studies in Child Welfare.

Address correspondence to the authors at the School of Social Work, University of Minnesota, 105 Peters Hall, 1404 Gortner Avenue, St. Paul, MN 55108.

[Haworth co-indexing entry note]: "Career Paths and Contributions of Four Cohorts of IV-E Funded MSW Child Welfare Graduates." Robin, Sandra C., and C. David Hollister. Co-published simultaneously in *Journal of Health & Social Policy* (The Haworth Press, Inc.) Vol. 15, No. 3/4, 2002, pp. 53-67; and: *Evaluation Research in Child Welfare: Improving Outcomes Through University-Public Agency Partnerships* (ed: Katharine Briar-Lawson, and Joan Levy Zlotnik) The Haworth Press, Inc., 2002, pp. 53-67. Single or multiple copies of this article are available for a fee from The Haworth Document Delivery Service [1-800-HAWORTH, 9:00 a.m. - 5:00 p.m. (EST). E-mail address: getinfo@haworthpressinc.com].

53

KEYWORDS. Social work education, Title IV-E, training funds, child welfare training, career development

INTRODUCTION

The federal government has contributed to the support of social work education for over forty years (Austin, Antonyappan & Leighninger, 1996). During the last decade the federal government has provided funds through Title IV-E of the Social Security Act to schools of social work to provide professional education in child welfare. An important purpose of this funding is to help counteract the trend in many states and counties toward the deprofessionalization of public child welfare work (Leighninger and Ellet, 1998; Briar-Lawson & Wiesen, 1999). The intended outcomes of IV-E programs typically include improved quality of public services to children and families and increased professional credibility of child welfare staff (Risley-Curtiss, McMurtry, Smith, Tobin, & Faddis, 1995). Through IV-E funding schools of social work have been encouraged to strengthen curricula in child welfare and to recruit social work students who will work in public child welfare following graduation.

Given the substantial funding occurring through Title IV-E, it is important that outcomes of IV-E funded programs be assessed. However, relatively few studies of IV-E outcomes have been published (Hopkins, Mudrick & Rudolph, 1999), nor has much been reported about the impacts of IV-E training on worker's career development. Do those social workers trained with IV-E funds stay in child welfare? Zlotnik and Cornelius (2000) note that "given the overall movement of social workers across practice fields, examining the career paths of these students supported by Title IV-E funds is an important trend to follow" (p. 13). The present article seeks to help fill this gap by presenting findings from a study of the career paths of four cohorts of IV-E funded MSW graduates of the child welfare specialization in one school of social work.

Background

Title IV-B and Title IV-E of the Social Security Act are the primary sources of federal funding for public child welfare services. The purpose of Title IV, Part E of the Social Security Act, "Federal Payments for Foster Care and Adoption Assistance," is to enable each state to provide foster care, transitional independent living programs, and adoption assistance for children with special needs (Social Security Act, 1980). Appropriations are authorized each fiscal year for states to provide these programs and services. In order to develop and enhance public agency worker's abilities to provide these programs and services for vulnerable children and families Title IV-E training entitlement monies are made available by the Child Welfare and Adoption Assistance Act of 1980, P.L. 96-272 (Zlotnik & Cornelius, 2000). The federal match for Title IV-B and Title IV-E is 75% to 25% non-federal dollars. Funds can be used to support both graduate and undergraduate training in child welfare in schools of social work.

This federal effort to professionalize child welfare practice has resulted in many partnerships between universities and public agencies across the country (Hopkins, Mudrick & Rudolph, 1999; Council on Social Work Education, 1997; Briar-Lawson & Wiesen, 1999). The federal government has supported this goal by spending millions of dollars annually for Title IV-E training (Zlotnik & Cornelius, 2000). When students receive IV-E funding to support their social work education, they are required to seek employment in child welfare in a public (county or state) agency upon graduation. The intended beneficiaries of this investment in social work-educated social workers are the children and families served through child protection, foster care and adoption programs.

One example of a university-public agency collaboration is the partnership between the University of Minnesota and the Minnesota Department of Human Services, which established the Center for Advanced Studies in Child Welfare (CASCW) within the School of Social Work. The partnership is now in its eighth year. It was initially established with the help of the Bush Foundation of Minnesota, which put up much of the 25% matching funds required to secure the 75% federal funding. The primary goals were to increase the cultural and ethnic diversity of social workers in public child welfare and to increase the cultural competence of all social workers in child welfare.

CASCW was established with Title IV-E funds through the Minnesota Department of Human Services to bring "the University of Minnesota together with county and state social services in a public-private partnership dedicated to improving the lives of high-risk families and children" (CASCW brochure, 2000). A major goal of CASCW is "to prepare graduate students to work in public social services with advanced preparation for the complex issues facing child welfare services" (CASCW brochure, 2000). One strategy for achieving this goal has been the development of a curriculum that prepares child welfare professionals with a family preservation focus that is sensitive to cultural and ethnic diversity. A second strategy has been the recruitment and admission each year of an ethnically diverse cohort of graduate students into the child welfare specialization and the provision of substantial financial support to them through the IV-E funded Child Welfare Scholars Program.

The Child Welfare Scholars Program is designed to diversify the staffing patterns of public child welfare services and to reinforce the development of an advanced professional staff to serve families and children at risk. Since its establishment in 1992, 212 students have been awarded IV-E scholarships. Close to sixty percent of these students have been students of color. To be chosen as a Child Welfare Scholar students must have demonstrated evidence of commitment and ability to be educated and employed in the field of child welfare; evidence of competency in, and commitment to, culturally sensitive practice with ethnic minorities, diverse communities, underserved populations, and people not of the applicant's own racial, ethnic, or cultural identification; and be a citizen of the United States or a permanent resident. The award is contingent upon satisfactory completion of the School's requirements, the availability of funding, and the maintenance of at least a 3.0 overall grade point average in graduate coursework. The Child Welfare Scholars are required to have at least one field placement in a county or state child welfare unit, and, upon graduating, to attain employment in child welfare in a public (county or state) agency (or if such is not available, to attain employment in another child welfare or school setting), and to commit to such employment for a period of time equal to the length of grant support, month for month.

METHOD

As part of an effort to assess the extent to which IV-E training has had an impact on the field of child welfare, we sought to ascertain the extent to which the IV-E MSW graduates had remained engaged in child welfare following the completion of their employment obligations to the IV-E program. The following research questions guided the study:

- What proportion of the Child Welfare Scholars in fact became employed in child welfare following graduation?
- For those Child Welfare Scholars employed in child welfare following graduation, what proportion worked in public child welfare settings vs. child welfare settings under private auspices?
- What proportion of the Child Welfare Scholars remained employed in child welfare following completion of their employment obligation?
- To what extent following graduation have Child Welfare Scholars provided leadership or made special contributions to the field of child welfare?

- Are there discernable patterns of job changes in the career paths of Child Welfare Scholars?
- For those Child Welfare Scholars who have left the field of child welfare, what work are they doing now, and what were their reasons for leaving child welfare?

Two sources of data were utilized–the records kept by CASCW on Child Welfare Scholar's post-MSW employment experience and a mailed questionnaire designed to ascertain aspects of graduate's careers not recorded in the CASCW database, such as specific job responsibilities or special contributions or leadership they may have provided.

The CASCW database records several sources of data submitted by the graduates, including both job-seeking efforts as well as post-MSW positions secured. Graduates are asked to submit a form that documents their acquisition of approved child welfare employment consistent with the Memorandum of Agreement signed by the student and the School of Social Work. Additionally, graduates were mailed a form in fall of 1999 requesting updated employment information. Not all 73 graduates in the first four cohorts responded with updated information, resulting in different "dates of last entry" for their employment information. Also, at their own initiative, graduates may update employment information by making an entry at the CASCW Web site. Approximately 10 graduates have done this.

Some of the information needed for the current study is not collected in the CASCW database. A questionnaire was, therefore, mailed to the Child Welfare Scholars who graduated in 1993, 1994, 1995, and 1996 to ascertain additional information about the extent to which their post-MSW career had been engaged with child welfare services. Respondents were asked about the amount of time they had worked in child welfare prior to beginning the MSW program; their positions following graduation; the development of their careers, including any special contributions they have made to the field of child welfare; and (for those who had left child welfare) their reasons for leaving the field. Although there are also later cohorts of IV-E graduates from this same program, the earlier cohorts were selected for this study, so that graduate's careers would have had at least a four-year period of opportunity for career development. Those in the earliest (1993) cohort had seven years of post-MSW career development at the time of the survey. Questionnaires were mailed to 71 of the 73 graduates in the four cohorts (the current addresses of two graduates were unattainable). Of the 71 surveyed, 32 responded (a 45% response rate). Three questionnaires were returned as undeliverable; more recent addresses could not be located for these graduates.

The characteristics of the four full cohorts and the survey respondents are shown in Table 1. The survey sample is quite representative of the four cohorts as a whole.

RESULTS

Initial Post-MSW Position of IV-E Graduates

The Four Full Cohorts

Of the 73 child welfare scholars graduating from 1993-1996, seventy-one, or 97%, became employed in child welfare. These graduates were employed in public social services, social work positions in private non-profit agencies, school social work positions, and social work positions in tribal social services. Two of the graduates secured employment in public social services but did not fulfill their employment obligation. Two other graduates accepted positions in private agencies, but there are no data on whether they completed their employment obligation. One graduate took a position unrelated to child welfare, and data are missing on one other graduate. For those graduates who completed their employment obligation the time they stayed in child welfare ranged from 8 months to 7 years (at date of last entry). Thus, of the 73 graduates in the four full cohorts, 66% (48) became employed in public child welfare; 18% (13) in private child welfare; 11% (8) in public schools and 3% (2) in tribal social services. One graduate was employed in a non-child welfare position and data on one graduate were unavailable.

Survey Respondents

All 32 of the respondents initially sought positions in public child welfare, as required by the IV-E grant. All 32 were successful in securing an initial position related to child welfare, although not all of the initial positions were in public child welfare agencies. The types of positions initially secured following graduation are shown in Table 2. Twenty of the 32 respondents (62.5%) were initially employed directly by a county social services department, either in child protection or in other IV-E related child welfare work. Eight (25%) of the other respondents found their first employment in private, non-profit child welfare agencies that contract with a public department of social services. Two others (6%) went initially into school social work. One of the remaining two respondents went into an administrative position in child welfare with state government and the other took a hospital-based social work position that dealt

TABLE 1. Characteristics of Four Full Cohorts and Survey Respondents

	Four Full Cohorts (N = 73)		Survey Respondents (N = 32)	
1. Mean Age	39.1		43.5	
	N	%	*N*	%
2. Gender				
Female	60	82%	26	81%
Male	13	18%	5	16%
Unavailable Data	0	0%	1	3%
	73	100%	32	100%
3. Ethnicity				
African American	15	20%	7	22%
American Indian	8	11%	1	3%
Asian American	6	8%	2	6%
European American	28	38%	19	60%
Multi-Ethnic	4	6%	2	6%
Unavailable Data	12	17%	1	3%
	73	100%	32	100%
4. MSW Plan				
Full Program	57	78%	25	78%
Advanced Standing	12	16%	7	22%
No File	4	6%	0	0%
	73	100%	32	100%
5. Year Completed Program				
1993	11	15%	5	16%
1994	20	27%	11	34%
1995	16	22%	5	16%
1996	26	36%	11	34%
	73	100%	32	100%
6. Experience in Child Welfare Prior to Entering MSW Program				
None			10	31%
1-2 years			8	25%
3-6 years	Not		6	19%
7-9 years	Ascertained		1	3%
10+ years			7	22%
			32	100%

TABLE 2. Initial Positions Secured by IV-E Graduates

	Four Full Cohorts (N = 73)		Survey Respondents (N = 32)	
	N	%	N	%
Child Welfare/Child Protection, County Agency	48	66%	20	62.5%
Child Welfare, Private Non-Profit Agency	13	18%	8	25.0%
School Social Work, Public School	8	11%	2	6.2%
Tribal Social Services	2	3%	0	0.0%
State Administration, Child Welfare	0	0%	1	3.1%
Hospital Social Work/Adolescent Mental Health	0	0%	1	3.1%
Non-Child Welfare	1	1%	0	0.0%
Unavailable Data	1	1%	0	0.0%
	73	100%	32	99.9%

with adolescent mental health. If the last two are included, then it can be said that all 32 (100%) of the respondents secured an initial position that involved them in IV-E related child welfare work directly or indirectly supported by public funds.

Retention of IV-E Graduates in Child Welfare

The Four Full Cohorts

At the date of last entry, 93% of the four cohorts of MSW graduates continued to be employed in child welfare. Table 3 summarizes retention data for these IV-E graduates.

Survey Respondents

We also analyzed the survey data, even though they describe a subset of the four full cohorts, because doing so provided current information on all those who responded. At the time of the survey, four to seven year's time had elapsed in the respondent's careers since their MSW graduation. Some graduates had remained in their initial positions; others had advanced within the same agency; and others had moved to positions in other agencies. Table 4 summarizes the changes that had occurred for these 32 respondents. Most had held only one or two positions since graduation. In those few instances where more than two positions had been held, only the initial and the last position were compared.

TABLE 3. Retention of IV-E Graduates in Child Welfare (At Date of Last Entry)

Of the 73 graduates, 68 (93%) continued to be employed in child welfare:

- 38 (52%) were in public child welfare positions
- 14 (19%) held child welfare positions in private agencies
- 7 (10%) were employed in a school setting
- 2 (3%) were employed in tribal social services
- 3 (4%) changed auspices of employment from public child welfare to a school or private agency setting
- 2 (3%) moved from a private agency into a public child welfare position
- 1 (1%) changed from a school setting to a private agency
- 1 (1%) changed from public to private and then back to public

Of the 73 graduates, 4 (6%) left the field of child welfare after completing their employment obligation:

- 2 left the field of social work
- 1 became a housing advocate
- 1 left to work with adults in the school system

For one (1%) of the graduates, there were no available data.

Table 4 indicates that the graduates responding had moved around a certain amount within the field of child welfare, broadly defined, but that almost all of them at the time of the survey still remained in some aspect of child welfare. At the time of the survey all but three of the 32 IV-E graduates responding were continuing to work in some aspect of child welfare, if school social work is included as a part of child welfare. (Five of the 32 graduates had started or moved into school social work.) Moreover, twelve of the thirty-two (38%) had clearly experienced promotions or advancement in their agencies. Others had changed agencies and it was sometimes difficult to tell if the change represented an advancement in responsibilities.

The three respondents who had left child welfare had taken other positions, one in adult developmental disabilities, one in library and information science, and one as homemaker and mother. Even these graduates indicated that their child welfare training was useful in their present work, for example, the developmental disabilities worker noted that he or she often works with client's families, and the library worker was in charge of the child welfare, social work, and sociology collections.

TABLE 4. Career Paths of the Survey Respondents

Of the 20 graduates whose initial employment was in county child welfare or child protection:

- 5 remained in their initial positions
- 7 advanced to other public child welfare or child protection positions
- 4 moved to positions in private child welfare
- 1 changed to work with adult developmentally disabled clients
- 1 changed to school social work
- 1 moved out of social work to library and information science (where she is "involved in selection of social work, child welfare, and sociology materials for the library collection" and also identifies and designs "content for a website aimed at family welfare and advocacy.")
- 1 ceased working after 41 months in child protection work to be "at home with my children"

Of the 8 graduates whose initial employment was in child welfare in private, non-profit agencies:

- 3 advanced to other positions in private child welfare agencies
- 2 moved to child protection work in county agencies
- 2 moved to school social work
- 1 moved to a state government position involving planning and training for child maltreatment prevention, child/youth suicide prevention, and fetal alcohol syndrome prevention

Of the two whose initial employment was in school social work:

- 1 remained in school social work
- 1 advanced into a combined administration/counseling position in a public alternative school

Of the two remaining respondents:

- the one in state administration of child welfare remained in that position
- the hospital social worker moved into a school social work position

---

Reasons for Leaving the Field

Several reasons were given by the three graduates who left the field, including "safety issues and stress" of child protection work, "better opportunities" in the new field, and a desire to be at home full time with her children. (One other graduate, who had moved from a frontline child protection worker to a training position in child protection, noted that "burnout in child protection" was the reason for the move.)

Contributions to Child Welfare

In the survey, graduates were asked to identify any special contributions and/or leadership they had provided to the field of child welfare since receiving the MSW degree. Responses to these open-ended questions were reviewed to see if any clusters of similar activities could be discerned. Seventeen different categories of contributions and leadership were identified. These are displayed in Table 5.

DISCUSSION

The findings from the database on the career paths of the four full cohorts of IV-E MSW graduates indicate that a very high proportion of them (66%) became employed in public child welfare upon graduation. If child welfare agencies under contract with county child welfare organizations and other child welfare settings are included, the figure is still higher (97%). This high proportion, of course, should be expected, because the graduates received substantial financial support for their MSW study and were obligated to accept employment in child welfare upon graduation for a period equal to the amount of time they received support.

Of greater interest is the question as to whether the IV-E graduates *remained* employed in child welfare after they had completed their obligations. Here again, we found that as of the last date of entry, 93% of the four full cohorts continued to be employed in child welfare and that 52% were continuing to work in public child welfare services. These data were corroborated by the survey data, which showed (for those responding) that fully 91% were continuing in child welfare as of May 2000. Thus, at least for these four cohorts, the vast majority of the graduates receiving IV-E funding have remained engaged in child welfare social work, well beyond the minimum required by the employment obligation. Moreover, almost all of the survey respondents reported significant contributions to leadership in child welfare, in such areas as planning, program development, administration, training, policy advocacy, ethical practice and research. These highly professionalized activities have a larger impact on the field of child welfare, extending beyond their co-workers, their clients and the immediate agency milieu.

There were no discernable patterns of job changes. A few who initially were employed in public child welfare moved into child welfare agencies under private auspices and some into school social work. But some of those initially in private child welfare also later moved into public child welfare. Interestingly, most graduates tended to stay in the agency of their initial employment. Only a

TABLE 5. Leadership and Special Contributions to the Field as Identified by Survey Respondents

Category	N[a]	Illustrative Examples
Administration	3	• "Moved as I wanted into administration and policy." • "Moved to administration."
Advocacy	7	Advocacy for: • minority children, especially those covered under ICWA • children and families • "Discuss issues of color with the Office of Civil Rights."
Consulting	2	• "Consulting work in the areas of collaboration, revenue enhancement and child welfare policy."
Cultural Competency	7	• "Help others and educate other professionals on issues involving children of color." • "My colleagues have great respect for my perceptions about families of color ...."
Grant Development and Fundraising	7	• "Instrumental in securing a multi-million dollar grant." • "Special project that I helped get funded for at risk families." • "I was able to pull in federal researchers and dollars to enhance a state-wide plan to address fetal alcohol syndrome." • "Instrumental in finding funding to provide in-school case management services to IV-E children."
Influencing Practice/Services Promoting Ethical Practice	12	• "I brought new sets of ideas and views while working with our families." • "Challenging the status quo and working to fight oppression as often as I can." • "Discussions during CP permanency retreats on improving practice and accessibility, including availability of services for parents and children."
Planning	4	• "Served on many strategic planning committees." • "Lead statewide planning in suicide prevention, resulting in legislative report and state plan."
Playwright/Theatre—for Community Outreach	1	• "I have continued to work with groups of teenagers (in a volunteer capacity) to write and produce plays performed locally for outreach to the community. Plays have included these issues: depression, suicide, domestic abuse ...."

TABLE 5 (continued)

Policy Leadership	4	• Leadership in policy efforts at the county and state levels • "Passage of legislation for pilot universal home visiting project in Minnesota."
Professional Associations	2	Leadership positions in: • Minnesota Social Service Association • Minnesota Chapter of Black Social Workers Association
Program Development	7	• "Took a program that was not adequately serving families and turned it into a responsive client centered program." • "Program improvements with children's services."
Research & Information Systems	4	• "Moved into greater responsibility (over a period of time) in the area of information systems and research evaluation." • "Work on the computer committee."
Statewide and Interagency Task Forces and Boards	4	• Representation and leadership on task forces and boards
Supervision	2	• Supervision of staff
Teaching	4	• Adjunct teaching faculty in undergraduate BSW program • Served as field instructor for social work interns
Team Building/Collaboration	10	• "Collaborative committee with medical center staff regarding child safety procedures." • "Part of a committee to enhance cultural diversity and awareness in our county. Did a county-wide project with a team to promote this work." • "Development of family service collaborative."
Training	9	• "Provide monthly training for pediatric residents regarding child protection reporting." • "Planned four training sessions related to Native American Social Work Issues which was attended by social service and child welfare professionals from both the public and private sectors." • "Presented training on kinship care and kinship placement to social service and legal professionals."

[a] N represents the number of respondents who identified leadership and/or special contributions in this category. N is larger than 32 due to multiple responses by respondents.

few graduates left the field of child welfare, and there was no consistent reason given by them for doing so.

Limitations

Caution is needed in generalizing from the findings. First, the data obtained from the records are from the first four cohorts of the school's graduates. It is possible, though perhaps unlikely, that the career patterns of later cohorts changed somewhat with changes in the environment. Second, the response rate for the survey was 45%. A possibility exists that the graduates who responded tended to be those who had provided greater than average leadership and contributions to the field. Graduates not responding to the survey may have been those who think their contributions have not been significant or that they have not been leaders in the field. Of course, the presence of social work-educated social workers in public child welfare is in itself a substantial contribution to the field and to the federal goal of professionalizing public child welfare services. Third, it would be useful to also collect data from supervisors and colleagues concerning the graduate's professional contributions and leadership; the data we have are self-reported. Fourth, all of the data are from the IV-E education program in just one school of social work. Other school's IV-E graduates may have had different career paths and experiences.

CONCLUSION

Through making Title IV-E training funds available to social work education programs, the federal government has made a substantial investment in, and commitment to, increasing the number of social work-educated social workers providing public child welfare services and, by doing so, to improving the quality of services to vulnerable children and families. This study suggests that the taxpayers are receiving good value for their money. The vast majority of graduates funded by IV-E training dollars became employed in and stayed in child welfare social work, with a high proportion staying in public child welfare services. These social work-educated social workers are actively involved in shaping the practice, policies and administration of child welfare services, and are thereby contributing to the federal goal of reprofessionalizing child welfare.

REFERENCES

Austin, M., Antonyappan, J. & Leighninger, L. (1996). Federal support for social work education: Section 707 of the 1967 Social Security Act amendments. *Social Service Review, 70* (1), 83-97.
Briar-Lawson, K., & Wiesen, M. (1999). Effective partnership models between state agencies, the university, and community service providers. In *1999 Child Welfare*

Training Symposium: Changing paradigms of child welfare practice: Responding to opportunities and challenges (pp. 73-86). Washington, D.C.: U.S. Department of Health and Human Services.

Center for Advanced Studies in Child Welfare. (2000). *Informational Brochure.* Saint Paul, MN.

Council on Social Work Education. (1997). *Preparing the workforce for family-centered practice: Social work education and public human services partnerships.* Alexandria, VA: author.

Hopkins, K. M., Murdock N. R. & Rudolph, C. S. (1999). Impact of university/agency partnerships in child welfare on organizations, workers, and work activities. *Child Welfare,* 78 (6), 749-773.

Leighninger, L., & Ellet, A. (1998, March). *Deprofessionalization in child welfare: Historical analysis and implications for social work education.* Paper presented at the Council on Social Work Education 44th Annual Meeting, Orlando, FL.

Risley-Curtiss, C., McMurty, S., Smith, E., Tobin, J., & Faddis, R. (1995, March). *Developing collaborative child welfare educational programs using Title IV-E funds.* Paper presented at the Council on Social Work Education 41st Annual Meeting, San Diego, CA.

Social Security Act, Title IV, *Part E-Federal Payments for Foster Care and Adoption Assistance,* §470, 42 U.S.C. 670. (1980).

Zlotnik, J. L., & Cornelius, L. F. (2000). Preparing social work students for child welfare careers: The use of Title IV-E training funds in social work education. *The Journal of Baccalaureate Social Work,* 5(2), 1-14.

Child Welfare Knowledge Transmission, Practitioner Retention, and University-Community Impact: A Study of Title IV-E Child Welfare Training

Kristin A. Gansle, PhD
Alberta J. Ellett, PhD

SUMMARY. This paper describes the implementation of a Title IV-E child welfare training program in Louisiana. A collaborative arrangement between the state child welfare agency and seven state university social work programs provides for student monetary stipends in return for child welfare training and work as public child welfare employees upon graduation. On a test of child welfare knowledge, students in MSW and BSW programs scored higher following child welfare training; BSW

Kristin A. Gansle is Assistant Professor, School of Social Work, Louisiana State University.

Alberta J. Ellett is Assistant Professor, University of Georgia School of Social Work.

Address correspondence to: Kristin A. Gansle, Assistant Professor, School of Social Work, Louisiana State University, 311 Huey P. Long Field House, Baton Rouge, LA 70803 (E-mail: kgansle@lsu.edu).

The authors wish to express their sincere thanks to all of the university faculty and agency supervisors and employees who have participated in this project, and to George H. Noell for his editorial assistance.

[Haworth co-indexing entry note]: "Child Welfare Knowledge Transmission, Practitioner Retention, and University-Community Impact: A Study of Title IV-E Child Welfare Training." Gansle, Kristin A., and Alberta J. Ellett. Co-published simultaneously in *Journal of Health & Social Policy* (The Haworth Press, Inc.) Vol. 15, No. 3/4, 2002, pp. 69-88; and: *Evaluation Research in Child Welfare: Improving Outcomes Through University-Public Agency Partnerships* (ed: Katharine Briar-Lawson, and Joan Levy Zlotnik) The Haworth Press, Inc., 2002, pp. 69-88. Single or multiple copies of this article are available for a fee from The Haworth Document Delivery Service [1-800-HAWORTH, 9:00 a.m. - 5:00 p.m. (EST). E-mail address: getinfo@haworthpressinc.com].

student stipend recipients made greater gains than non-recipients when controlling for initial scores. MSW students' results appear to approach significance; they may not be significant due to low power of the statistical analysis. Child welfare agency retention of the stipend student graduates is considered good by the agency. *[Article copies available for a fee from The Haworth Document Delivery Service: 1-800-HAWORTH. E-mail address: <getinfo@haworthpressinc.com> Website: <http://www.HaworthPress.com> © 2002 by The Haworth Press, Inc. All rights reserved.]*

KEYWORDS. Child welfare, Title IV-E, program evaluation, de-professionalization

INTRODUCTION

Employing and retaining competent employees is critical to the success of any organization. In fields such as public child welfare, it is especially important due to the potentially life-altering effects of workers' decisions on children and their families. The effective and benevolent execution of child welfare policies and directives is necessarily tied to the skills of child welfare workers; the quality of services in child welfare can be only as high as the quality of the professionals who provide them (Ewalt, 1991).

Since its inception, the U.S. Department of Health and Human Services (DHHS) has recognized the need for skilled staff in child welfare and has funded continuing education stipends for public child welfare workers to develop competence in child welfare practice (Ellett, Ellett, Kelley, & Noble, 1996). The Social Security Act of 1935 contained provisions for providing higher education to individuals employed in child welfare. However, over time, inadequate funding, increased social problems, and increased governmental mandates to provide supplementary services without concomitant financial support have greatly countered these efforts to enhance professional proficiencies in child welfare.

For example, the Child Abuse Prevention and Treatment Act of 1974 required all states to create child abuse and neglect reporting systems (Costin, Karger, & Stoesz, 1996; Pecora, Whittaker, & Maluccio, 1992). This legislation increased the need for child welfare workers to manage paperwork, investigate reports of child abuse and neglect, and provide services in founded cases of child abuse and neglect. Furthermore, reported cases of child abuse and neglect tripled from 669,000 in 1976 to 2,086,000 in 1986 (Child Welfare Stat Book, 1993) and doubled again from 1,420,000 in 1986 to 2,810,000 in 1993, with the number of seriously injured children quadrupling from 141,700 in 1986 to 565,00 in 1993 (DHHS, 1996). Despite the increased pressure on the system, funding to state child welfare agencies did not increase proportionally.

By the early 1990s, appropriations for Title XX for child abuse and neglect represented only half the value established in 1974 (Costin et al., 1996).

The past quarter-century clearly has brought many changes in the system. With the increase in the demands on social services systems (Child Welfare Stat Book, 1993) as a result of legislation, the increase in the needs of families due to factors such as chemical dependency, and the complexities associated with caring for families and their children, there has also been a noticeable decline in the skills of child welfare workers due to declassification. As used here, this declassification (Costin et al., 1996; Lewandowski, 1998), or de-professionalization of positions refers to reducing or eliminating the minimum educational qualifications, particularly degrees in social work, for positions in public child welfare. In the 1960s, the expected credential of child welfare professionals was an MSW (Abramczyk, 1994). Today, however, due to the increased demands on the system and an inadequately trained workforce, these requirements have been relaxed. In many states, a high school diploma or a bachelor's degree (not necessarily in the social sciences) is the entry-level job requirement. This de-professionalization, combined with job demands that have only increased and a lack of adequate professional preparation, has fostered high employee turnover (Ellett et al., 1996; Pecora et al., 1992). Russell and Hornby (1987) reported 15% turnover and vacancy among child welfare positions in states with bachelor's or MSW requirements, while the rate of turnover and vacancy in states with no degree requirement is 23%.

In discussing de-professionalization, Costin and colleagues (Costin et al., 1996, p. 158) state that with de-professionalization "there is the assumption of the interchangeableness of bachelor's degrees, the reorganization of jobs to reduce educational requirements, the substitution of experience for education, [and] the nonrecognition of the exclusivity of bachelor's and master's degrees in social work." The employment of well-meaning, but untrained individuals who are expected to carry out complex policies and to deliver services to the nation's most needy and troubled population has not maintained the quality of the services delivered to clients of departments of social services. When these employees who often do not have social work degrees, and who often are not adequately trained to provide social work services, fail to protect children from severe abuse or neglect, these cases are often sensationalized in the media. Even though the implicated workers often do not hold social work degrees, they are referred to as "social workers" (Costin et al., 1996; Pecora et al., 1992). The negative publicity associated with such events tends to tarnish the reputation of social workers and can prevent adequate resources from being afforded them to do their jobs well. In order to preserve the ability of social work to serve its clients, as well as the health and welfare of the profession, it is of the utmost importance that we hire qualified employees who have the requisite skills and knowledge necessary for child welfare assignments and who can contribute to the organization's ability to carry out its mission and statutory mandates.

There are factors that contribute to the retention of a professional and well-trained workforce. The literature has suggested several factors that are likely to increase child welfare employee retention: credentialing and licensing that represent expertise in the field, symbolic recognition of workers' achievements as well as tangible rewards and promotional opportunities, increased "people work over paper work," and improved work environments (Helfgott, 1991; Jayaratne & Chess, 1984; Pecora et al., 1989; Reagh, 1994; Rycraft, 1994; Vinokur-Kaplan, 1991). This paper reviews Louisiana's use of IV-E funds to effect changes in the preparation of workers in order to increase skills and achieve better retention of competent employees.

Louisiana's Child Welfare Training and Curriculum Development Project is currently comprised of the state child welfare agency and the seven state universities that grant social work degrees in Louisiana. These organizations use IV-E funds to provide supports necessary to enhance child welfare employee preparation, recruitment, selection, and retention. This program is based on the premise that hiring competent social workers will lead to increased caseworker success and improved client outcomes.

The Child Welfare Preparation Program

The Louisiana Department of Social Services, Office of Community Services (OCS), is the public child welfare agency responsible for child protection, services to abusive/neglectful parents and their families, foster care, adoption, and the recruitment, training, and certification of foster and adoptive families. This agency is state and federally funded and administered with a central state office in Baton Rouge, in addition to offices in nearly every parish in Louisiana and each of ten regions.

Due to the changing context of child welfare practice, schools and departments of social work have begun to work more closely with state child welfare agencies. One critical need they have addressed is the adequate professional preparation of workers to provide quality services to children and families. With funds provided by the Adoption Assistance and Child Welfare Act of 1980, OCS and seven Louisiana university schools and departments of social work developed a program for pre-service education, employment, and support of child welfare professionals. The purpose of the program is to recruit, educate, and prepare graduates for competent practice in child welfare to enhance professionalism within OCS. The goals of the preparation program are many. First, individuals competent in child welfare practice will be graduated from our state universities' social work programs. Second, employees in public child welfare will be attracted and maintained. Third, competent OCS employees will be trained and retained. Fourth, employees will focus on services for multi-problem families. Fifth, employees will maintain a philosophy of family-focused and child-centered intervention, so that they will move toward a family systems approach rather than an individual pathology approach. Sixth, collaborative efforts between Louisiana universities' schools and departments of social work and OCS will be established, maintained, and enhanced.

These programs include:

a. cooperative arrangements between OCS and seven universities,
b. student stipends,
c. revisions in university curriculum to include child welfare content,
d. supervised internships in public child welfare,
e. postgraduate employment with OCS, and
f. program evaluation. These are described in greater detail below.

Cooperative arrangements between OCS and seven universities. The decision was made by OCS to begin this program with one university, Louisiana State University (LSU), in the fall of 1993. This program served as a pilot as well as a field test of the program to identify problems and to incorporate adjustments and changes as indicated. The program was expanded in 1994 to Southern University, Southern University at New Orleans, and Northwestern State University. Southeastern Louisiana University and Northeast Louisiana University joined in 1995 and Grambling State University began their program in fall of 1997. This raised the number of MSW programs to two and BSW programs to six, thereby including all seven state universities with schools and departments of social work in Louisiana. Because the number of student stipends at each university is small, a decision was made to pool resources and develop one evaluation protocol to employ with each participating university. Contracts between the universities and OCS specify that in return for funds for student stipends and the addition of faculty hours for teaching, supervision, instructional materials, and related responsibilities, universities would, in conjunction with OCS staff, select students to participate in the stipend program, supervise their internships within OCS, and supervise the collection of data relevant to program evaluation.

Student stipends. Teams of university faculty and OCS internship supervisors interview students who apply to the program. Students selected for the program display a serious interest in working with children and families on a long-term basis. They present well and interviewers expect that they will succeed as child welfare workers. Students who are chosen are required to sign a legally binding agreement that specifies their responsibilities with respect to the program. They agree to study required child welfare coursework, complete their internships at OCS, and participate in an extensive evaluation in return for a stipend that has ranged from approximately $5,000 for BSW students to $7,000 for MSW students, depending on the university and the program in which the student is enrolled. In return for the year's stipend, students are required to work for OCS for one calendar year upon graduation from their program. The last requirement is contingent upon the availability of positions within the OCS system in Louisiana. Students who are offered employment but choose to work only part or none of their required year are expected to repay all or part of their stipend, depending on the amount of time they have worked for OCS.

Revisions in university child welfare curriculum. Prior to the implementation of the program, each university was responsible for developing a plan for and incorporating child welfare content into the BSW or MSW program curriculum. This content was provided in the form of a list of competencies that designers of the program expected proficient child welfare workers to acquire (available from the authors upon request). Universities were given some latitude with respect to how they chose to implement instruction toward child welfare competencies within their respective curricula. Some chose to offer separate child welfare courses; others chose to include child welfare content within the curricula of extant courses, thereby integrating child welfare information throughout the program curriculum. Programs are about equally split regarding how they chose to integrate child welfare content.

Supervised internships in public child welfare. Students are assigned to local OCS offices where they receive a few cases with which to work throughout the duration of their internship in concert with the assigned worker and supervisor. Some of the duties they are expected to perform with supervision include taking child abuse/neglect reports by telephone, writing social histories, writing court reports, participating in agency staffings, attending court hearings, working on life books with children, and accompanying workers in all programs in all aspects of their jobs.

Postgraduate employment with OCS. Stipend recipients file necessary application forms and interview for positions within OCS. If they are selected, they agree to work for OCS for a minimum of one calendar year. Students consent to delay employment with other agencies for two months following their graduation dates. If, within two months of graduation, no position is offered to a graduate of the program, the student is released from the contract and no funds are expected to be repaid. If the student is offered employment and declines the OCS employment offer or fails to graduate, a schedule is designed for the student to repay the stipend funds to the program. To date, no students have failed to graduate from the program.

Program evaluation. An integral part of the grant of Title IV-E funds to the recipient universities is the evaluation of the effects of the projects. This evaluation is underway to determine the progress of the universities toward the goals of the project. Variables measured include project participants' child welfare knowledge, the effectiveness of the program in preparing students for work with the Office of Community Services (OCS), and the staff retention rate of workers who began their careers with OCS as a result of this Title IV-E program.

METHOD

Participants

IV-E stipend students. From 1993 to summer 2000, there have been 174 students who have participated in the program. Seventy-two were in MSW programs and 102 in BSW programs. Five of the BSW students went on to become project participants in MSW programs in Louisiana, and are also included in the MSW total. For retention data, those students are considered only once, as part of the MSW group.

Students participating in IV-E project testing. Because two different analyses were completed (see below), two different sets of demographics are presented. There is some overlap in those data due to the nature of the analyses. Demographic data, including the mean age, ethnicities, genders of students, are presented in Tables 1 and 2.

Design

Students were chosen to participate in the stipend program following application, screening, and interview. Due to the lack of random assignment of participants in the evaluation to stipend and non-stipend groups, the program evaluation used a quasi-experimental design. The two factors included stipend group and administration (time).

Dependent Variables

Child welfare skills and knowledge. Although there were many possible indicators of competent child welfare practice for child welfare workers, similar measures were difficult to obtain for child welfare students. Students may not have had the requisite opportunities to practice their new skills with the feedback necessary to become proficient in these skills. In lieu of a direct assessment of skills, which was logistically impossible for project administrators to

TABLE 1. Demographic Data for IV-E Project Evaluation Participants Set I: 1994-1999

		MSW students	BSW students
stipend students	total number	48	90
	mean age	31.1 years	28.3 years
	African-Americans	21 (52.5%)	40 (51.9%)
	Caucasians	19 (47.5%)	36 (46.8%)
	women	34 (85%)	70 (89.7%)
	men	6 (15%)	8 (10.3%)
non-stipend students	total number	137	418
	age	29.8 years	26.8 years
	African-Americans	37 (28.0%)	199 (51.7%)
	Caucasians	88 (66.7%)	173 (44.5%)
	women	120 (90.9%)	342 (88.8%)
	men	12 (9.1%)	43 (11.2%)

Note: Total number represents all students participating in the evaluation. The balance of data represents information for those students who chose to report information.

TABLE 2. Demographic Data for IV-E Project Evaluation Participants Set II: 1996-1999

		MSW	BSW
stipend students	total number	35	66
	mean age	30.3 years	28.1 years
	African-Americans	21 (60.0%)	34 (52.3%)
	Caucasians	14 (40.0%)	30 (46.2%)
	women	30 (85.7%)	59 (89.4%)
	men	5 (14.3%)	7 (10.6%)
non-stipend students	total number	102	332
	age	30.4 years	26.8 years
	African-American	32 (31.4%)	177 (53.2%)
	Caucasians	65 (63.7%)	146 (43.8%)
	women	94 (82.2%)	292 (87.7%)
	men	8 (7.8%)	41 (12.3%)

Note: Total number represents all students participating in the evaluation. The balance of data represents information for those students who chose to report information.

complete, a paper-and-pencil test of child welfare knowledge was used to assess fundamental prerequisite knowledge for competent child welfare practice. No test of child welfare knowledge with demonstrated reliability and validity was available; consequently, a test was constructed to assess knowledge of child welfare-relevant topics. This test will be discussed in more detail below.

Child welfare knowledge. Child welfare knowledge is measured using the Louisiana Examination of Child Welfare Information (LECWI). The LECWI is an examination designed by the authors to evaluate child welfare knowledge. It is composed of questions on child welfare topics that have been contributed by the faculty and staff who administer the Title IV-E program at the various participating universities. The questions cover many topics, including child protection, family preservation and in-home services, foster care, adoption, foster/adoptive home recruitment and certification, permanency planning or "reasonable efforts," history of child welfare, policy, and other general child welfare competencies.

Some questions assess factual knowledge and some are designed to allow students to apply their knowledge. The latter questions usually present a vignette and ask students to choose the best course of action from four possible answers. Students' scores on various administrations of the LECWI were figured as a percentage of items answered correctly. The LECWI began with 53 items; since fall, 1996, the LECWI has contained 60 items.

Test construction. At the start of the IV-E project, a test of child welfare knowledge, then unnamed, was constructed. Each year since, all participating program's coordinators were asked to provide a sample of new questions for possible use on the LECWI. Questions are multiple choice with four possible choices. Each question has one correct answer.

An analysis of the items from the pre-test for the previous year has been completed each summer. Items that are too easy (greater than 90% of the students answer correctly), that have choices that no one uses, and that have a low item-total correlation were removed from the test or edited. Remaining items were kept for the new test. Depending on the number of questions that must be replaced, each participating university has equal representation in the questions that are replaced.

Reliability. For each year, all scores from the fall administration of the tests were submitted to a reliability analysis. A measure of internal consistency, Cronbach's Alpha, was calculated for each scale. Alpha can range between 0 and 1. Nunnally (1978) recommends that for research purposes, where there are not yet many data available in an area, an alpha of .7 or higher is acceptable. As the research matures, .8 is considered to be internally consistent. Table 3 provides the alphas for the LECWI scales by year.

Common items. To permit analyses across program years, two sets of items that were common across years were selected from the set of tests. First, the 21 items common to all tests were used in a set of analyses covering the complete program (Set I, years 1994-1999). Second, a set of 38 items common to the latest three program years (Set II, years 1996-1999) were employed in an additional set of analyses.

Retention rate. In addition, staff retention rate is a variable of major concern to child welfare agencies. This project examined the percentage of those program graduates who were still employed with the Office of Community Services after they had completed the requirements of their contract. This information was collected from the personnel division of the Office of Community Services in Louisiana.

Independent Variables

Participants in the project were students who enrolled in either a bachelor's or master's program in social work. Due to the differences in the program's student bodies, all analyses examine MSW program students and BSW program students separately.

Stipend group. This variable has two levels: students who receive a stipend and participate in the project and those who do not. It is important to bear in mind that the program is not static. It is constantly being revised and refined based on the experiences and reports of the participants, university faculty, and front-line internship supervisors. Aspects of the program that are common to all programs include a public child welfare internship and supervision, receipt of the stipend, study of required child welfare curriculum, and agreement to participate in evaluation of the program.

Time. Students who participate in testing do so prior to beginning their last year of their academic program and just prior to their graduation. This creates a pre-program and post-program administration of examinations.

TABLE 3. Alphas for LECWI Scales by Year of Stipend Program

year	n	number of items	α
1994-1995	53	53	.54
1995-1996	118	53	.63
1996-1997	148	60	.70
1997-1998	151	60	.79
1998-1999	192	60	.84

PROCEDURE

Prior to the beginning of the academic year, applications were solicited by the universities for stipends. University faculty and OCS supervisors chose stipend recipients collaboratively. In return for their stipend money, students sign agreements to study required child welfare content in their courses, to participate in a supervised internship in public child welfare, to participate in other activities designated by the university they attend, and to participate in evaluation of the program.

At the beginning of the stipend period, stipend students and their non-stipend classmates take the Louisiana Examination of Child Welfare Information and provide project administrators with a variety of demographic information. All information is kept confidential; no individual scores or information are released to any project or university personnel. The same data are collected at the end of the stipend period.

Data are collected throughout the State and analyzed as a group. IV-E stipend students are expected to participate in the evaluation of the program so that project administrators and funding agencies may be aware of program outcomes.

Analysis. Due to the fact that IV-E stipend students are selected based on exceptional academics and commitment to the field of child welfare, it is expected that their knowledge of child welfare would be greater than those who are not chosen. Therefore, where inferential statistics were appropriate, a Repeated Measures Analysis of Variance (RM ANOVA) was used. This repeated measures analysis controls for differences in pre-program scores of participant groups.

The major research question of this investigation involves how differences in stipend experiences affect the change in test scores over time. To this end, the repeated measures analyses of variance were run for the purpose of examining the significance of the interactions of the two main variables: stipend group (2 levels) by time (2 levels). These interactions answered the main research questions. Main effects of those independent variables are reported for completeness, but the research questions will be answered best by the significance of the interactions.

The degree to which program participants were retained by OCS was examined using a simple rate at which workers are retained following their requisite year of employment with the Agency. Rates are calculated for MSW and BSW IV-E program graduates.

RESULTS

Reliability of the LECWI

Examination of the data in Table 3 indicates that the Louisiana Examination of Child Welfare Information (LECWI) is becoming more reliable each year it is fine-tuned.

Retention Rate of IV-E Stipend Recipients

There have been 72 graduates of IV-E students from MSW programs. Of these 72 graduates, 60 (83%) were employed with OCS. Thirty-three (55% of those who were employed) were still employed with OCS as of March 1, 2000. Specific data regarding length of employment with OCS by stipend year are included in Table 4. There have been 97 graduates of IV-E students from BSW programs. This number does not include those IV-E program students who graduated from their BSW programs and went on to complete an MSW as a IV-E stipend recipient. Those students were included as part of the MSW program student group. Of these 97 graduates of BSW programs only, 32 (33%) were employed with OCS. Twenty-seven (84% of those who were employed) were still employed with OCS as of March 1, 2000. Specific data regarding length of employment with OCS by stipend year are included in Table 4.

LECWI Scores

LECWI scores were analyzed separately for MSW and BSW students, and for the 1994-1999 data (21 test items, Set I) and the 1996-1999 data (38 test items, Set II).

Set I. For MSW students, a Repeated Measures ANOVA revealed a significant effect for time, $F (1, 183) = 44.64$, $p < .0001$. The effects for stipend

TABLE 4. Length of Tenure of IV-E Program Graduates Work at Office of Community Services

program	stipend year	mean tenure in years	range of tenure in years		number of students
			minimum	maximum	
MSW	1998-1999	.7	.6	.8	4
	1997-1998	1.4	.12	1.8	9
	1996-1997	1.6	.14	2.8	10
	1995-1996	2.8	1.5	3.8	11
	1994-1995	3.4	.14	4.8	14
	1993-1994	4.3	1.5	5.8	12
BSW	1998-1999	1.0	.6	1.2	9
	1997-1998	1.0	.24	1.7	7
	1996-1997	2.4	.8	3.2	9
	1995-1996	3.2	2.6	4.2	4
	1994-1995	2.5	.33	5.2	3

group, F (1, 183) = 2.14, p = .15, and the interaction of group and time F (1, 183) = 0.30, p = .59, were not significant. Students' scores on the test of child welfare knowledge were significantly different before and after the program; however, stipend students did no better or worse than their non-stipend counterparts, and the stipend groups did not change differently over time. Please see Table 5 for the means and standard deviations, and Figure 1 for a graphic representation of these data.

For BSW students, a Repeated Measures ANOVA revealed a significant effect for time, F (1, 506) = 73.12, p < .001, for stipend group, F (1, 506) = 87.68, p < .001, and for the interaction of group and time F (1, 506) = 33.57, p < .001. Students' scores on the test of child welfare knowledge were significantly higher at the end of the academic year, stipend students did better than their non-stipend counterparts, and the stipend students' scores changed more than either of their non-stipend counterparts. Please see Table 5 for the means and standard deviations, and Figure 1 for a graphic representation of these data.

Set II. For MSW students, a Repeated Measures ANOVA revealed a significant effect for time, F (1, 135) = 16.12, p < .001. The effects for stipend group, F (1, 135) = 2.11, p = .15, and the interaction of group and time F (1, 135) = 2.13, p = .15, were not significant. Students' scores on the test of child welfare knowledge were significantly different before and after the program; however, stipend students did no better or worse than their non-stipend counterparts, and the stipend groups did not change differently over time. Please see Table 6 for the means and standard deviations, and Figure 2 for a graphic representation of these data.

For BSW students, a Repeated Measures ANOVA revealed a significant effect for time, F (1, 396) = 81.43, p < .001, for stipend group, F (1, 396) = 77.86, p < .001, and for the interaction of group and time F (1, 396) = 29.06, p < .001. Students' scores on the test of child welfare knowledge were significantly different before and after the program, stipend students did better than their non-stipend counterparts, and the stipend groups changed differently over

TABLE 5. Means and Standard Deviations of Set I, 21-Item LECWI Scores for Student Stipend Groups

| | stipend | | | | | non-stipend | | | | |
| | pre | | post | | | pre | | post | | |
program	M	SD	M	SD	N	M	SD	M	SD	N
MSW	64.8%	14.8	72.5%	14.9	48	61.8%	14.9	68.4%	17.1	137
BSW	59.1%	16.0	69.9%	16.1	90	49.1%	14.2	51.1%	14.7	419

FIGURE 1. Means of 21-Item LECWI Scores for Student Stipend Groups by Program

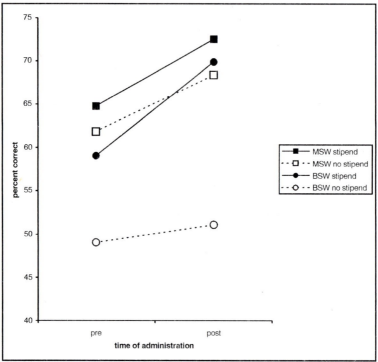

time. Please see Table 6 for the means and standard deviations, and Figure 2 for a graphic representation of these data.

DISCUSSION

LECWI as Indicator of Child Welfare Knowledge and Skills

The Louisiana Examination of Child Welfare Information appears to be an internally consistent measure. It has become more reliable each year it has been in development (according to Nunnally, 1978). Although no formal indices of validity have yet been collected, its content matches the areas of child welfare that university faculty in social work consider important to child welfare competence. Areas for further research and development of the LECWI include a more formal validity analysis and correlation of the examination with other indices of employee skill and proficiency.

TABLE 6. Means and Standard Deviations of Set II, 38-Item LECWI Scores for Student Stipend Groups

| | stipend | | | | | non-stipend | | | | |
| | pre | | post | | | pre | | post | | |
program	M	SD	M	SD	N	M	SD	M	SD	N
MSW	59.8%	13.2	66.2%	15.4	35	57.8%	13.9	60.8%	15.0	102
BSW	55.2%	66	65.3%	14.4	66	44.9%	12.2	47.5%	13.0	332

FIGURE 2. Means of 38-Item LECWI Scores for Student Stipend Groups by Program

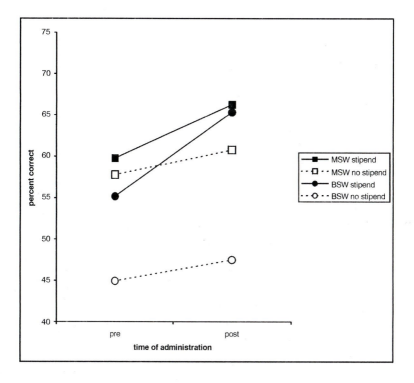

Retention Rate

During the six years for which data were analyzed for this paper, 83% of Louisiana's MSW IV-E program graduates and 33% of Louisiana's BSW IV-E program graduates were employed with the State public child welfare agency. For MSWs, 55% of those are still employed, and for BSWs, 84% of those are still employed. Prior to September 1996, OCS BSW students did not qualify for OCS entry-level positions because of Civil Service requirements regarding new hires. Consequently, none of the BSWs who were required to work for OCS in order to satisfy their contracts could be hired by the agency. Although this was known prior to the signing of contracts each year, it was expected that a compromise solution could be reached before that group of BSW stipend students had graduated from their respective programs and that those graduates could be employed by the agency. Although the OCS employment rate was seriously affected by Civil Service employment requirements, the decision was made to continue the IV-E project within BSW programs while work on a new job classification was underway.

This took much longer than expected. The agency now has a new job classification for BSWs graduating from this university child welfare preparation program. Since the commencement of hiring under this new job classification, the probability that program graduates will be hired is much improved. The retention rate for those hired is considered excellent by the agency. Retention data for MSW program graduates is not as encouraging. Although a greater proportion of MSW graduates have become employed with OCS, only 55% of those have chosen to stay to date. Anecdotally, many of those who leave use their skills with similar populations at other agencies; consequently, their training continues to have a positive impact on the community as a whole. Similar retention rates at OCS for new employees who are not graduates of the IV-E program are not tracked; however, a Louisiana statewide study has found turnover rates in the first three years of employment ran as high as 39% in urban offices (Ellett et al., 1996). It is a priority for future evaluation within OCS and the IV-E project that those data be tracked and become available for analysis so that program graduate's MSW and BSW retention rate may be compared to other OCS employees.

Although no data collection has yet been done in this area, MSW graduates of the program have expressed concern that the lack of professionally credentialed supervisors, and a lack of support for new OCS employees have made remaining with the agency difficult. They report that the pay continues to be too low and the work and bureaucracy professionally stifling. Program administrators are discussing the possibility of the universities providing additional support and training to child welfare workers throughout the State to attempt to ameliorate some of these concerns.

Child Welfare Knowledge

For the purpose of evaluating the effects of this program on student knowledge of child welfare-relevant topics, the primary question investigated using a multi-site collaboratively-developed examination of child welfare knowledge is whether students who are part of the group receiving the IV-E child welfare stipend for their work during their degree program perform better on this examination of child welfare knowledge than those who are not.

There are clear differences between the MSW and BSW groups. Results from the 21-item and 38-item versions of the examination seem similar. MSW students begin their programs with a greater fund of knowledge related to child welfare. MSW stipend students increase scores at about the same rate as non-stipend students. However, BSW students are a different matter. BSW stipend students appear to increase their scores to a much greater degree over time than their non-stipend counterparts. And, they increase those scores to a point where they exceed the scores of non-stipend MSW students.

There are several possibilities that might explain this phenomenon. MSW programs may be providing similar child welfare classroom experiences to all social work students, thereby increasing their knowledge. BSW programs may be providing more focused child welfare-specific courses or instruction to their IV-E program students. It is also possible that these differences are due to the greater differences between MSW and BSW students in general. There are fewer MSW than BSW students, and there is probably greater variability in academic skills among BSW students than among MSW students who have proceeded to study for an advanced degree. It is likely that the BSW students who are chosen for the stipend program are much better students than their peers. They may learn information at a greater rate than their peers, thereby creating a greater gap than the MSW stipend students do.

Another factor to consider is that there may not have been enough MSW stipend students included in the analysis. The interactions appeared to be approaching significance, and with a larger N, those effects may have been significant (Kraemer & Thiemann, 1987). Increases in the number of participants in the coming years may increase power and yield different results.

In any case, students in social work programs throughout the state, be they stipend recipients or not, are receiving some benefit in child welfare knowledge and skills from the instruction provided by faculty and supervisors through the universities.

The Big Picture

Work with children and families in child welfare is complex, and successful practice requires considerable development of professional skills. The child welfare preparation model described in this paper has consolidated the benefits of both higher education and on-the-job training with some encouraging results. This collaborative effort between seven state university schools and departments of social work and OCS to enhance the preparation of graduates for child welfare practice is now in its seventh year. Many adjustments and revisions in the program and evaluation had to be accommodated along the way. Some of these missteps and adjustments may be of interest to others considering or engaged in similar projects.

Identified Glitches and Solutions in the Program

The program was funded shortly before the start of its first academic year. With only a few weeks to start up, we were only able to do a paper review of student applicants and two of the six student stipend recipients dropped out. They were unclear about what child welfare work entailed, and were simply unsuited to work in child welfare. We now review applications, require three references (two faculty and one social worker), and conduct an interview jointly with faculty and local OCS staff together before making final selections. It has become evident that closer work with local staff who often provide the students' internship supervision and value their participation in selection of students who are future employees is important to assuring the success of the program.

We failed to recognize the value of an orientation to the overall project for stipend students the first year; they seemed lost about the scope of the program and their role therein. An annual orientation meeting has since provided students with an opportunity to hear more about the specifics of the program as well as to ask questions regarding employment and their contract responsibilities. There was some initial reluctance of local supervisors to supervise students, which dissipated when they were able to hire them. Now staff members volunteer to supervise students in this program, which also provides supervisors respect and status within their local offices.

Since the commencement of the program, it has become clear that internship supervisors are critical to the success of the program for the students. Consequently, they have received increased attention over time. Some funds are now set aside for continuing education. The IV-E projects have been expanded at the participating universities to include in-service training for those OCS supervisors who provide stipend recipients' internship supervision. These individuals are permitted to attend one national child welfare conference, which serves as both an incentive to mentor stipend students as well as to provide excellent training opportunities to stipend students.

Encouraging Results

As for any long-term project, evaluation is dynamic and ongoing. Data will continue to be collected over a period of years. Despite attempts to do so, OCS would not allow access to employee evaluations to see how graduates' job skills compared to others of similar length of employment. An instrument to evaluate employee performance is in the developmental phase.

Participating universities and OCS believe this program will help reverse the trend of de-professionalization and declassification to one of professionalization in public child welfare. As students are exposed to child welfare as a viable practice area, individuals who would not have otherwise considered employment in public child welfare now do. Other students who do not consider employment in public child welfare do consider what it would be like to work with child welfare clients in other social work settings, which improves services to child welfare clients.

As schools and departments of social work institutionalize child welfare into their curricula, many benefits, including recognition of child welfare as an important practice area, are realized. These collaborations may lead to an alliance with public child welfare agencies, and other social work associations and higher education to encourage Civil Service systems to require social work degrees for social work jobs within child welfare. Working with Civil Service to establish pay commensurate with education and better compensation will improve capacity to recruit MSW and BSW graduates into child welfare. Increasing the proportion of MSW and BSW staff in child welfare agencies will improve services to clients and may actually lead to an improved work environment.

The child welfare preparation program appears to be accomplishing its main goal: graduating individuals competent in child welfare practice. Feedback from supervisors of employed stipend recipients is that they are able to hit the ground running with cases much more quickly than other new hires. In addition, the new cooperative program enhances student enthusiasm for work in child welfare, university faculty members have significantly increased child welfare content in revised curricula, and anecdotally, student's positive evaluations of the program are increasing over time. With time, we hope the positive trend will only continue.

REFERENCES

Abramczyk, L. (1994). Should child welfare workers have an M.S.W.? In E. Gambrel & T. Stein (Eds.), *Controversial issues in child welfare* (pp. 174-786). Needham Heights, MA: Allyn & Bacon.

Adoption Assistance and Child Welfare Act of 1980, Pub. L. No. 96-272, §§ 101, 102.

Child Abuse Prevention and Treatment Act of 1974, Pub. L. No. 93-247.

Child maltreatment 1996: Reports from the states to the National Child Abuse and Neglect Data System. (1996). Washington, D.C.: U.S. Department of Health and Human Services.

The child welfare stat book. (1993). Washington, D.C.: Child Welfare League of America, Inc.

Costin, L., Karger, H., & Stoesz, D. (1996). *The politics of child abuse and neglect in America.* New York: Oxford Press.

Ellett, C., Ellett, A., Noble, D., & Kelley, B. (1996). Statewide study of child welfare personnel: Who leaves, who stays, who cares? Paper presented at CSWE 1996 Annual Program Meeting Washington, D.C.

Ewalt, P. (1991). The trends affecting recruitment and retention of social work staff in human services agencies. *Social Work, 36,* 214-217.

Helfgott, K. (1991). *Staffing the child welfare agency: Recruitment and retention.* Washington, D.C.: Child Welfare League of America Inc.

Jayaratne, S., & Chess, W. (1984). Job satisfaction, burnout, and turnover: A national study. *Social Work, 29,* 448-453.

Kraemer, H. C., & Thiemann, S. (1987). *How many subjects? Statistical power analysis in research.* Newbury Park, CA: Sage.

Lewandowski, C. A. (1998). Retention outcomes of a public child welfare long-term training program. *Professional Development: The International Journal of Continuing Social Work Education, 1,* 38-46.

Nunnally, J. C. (1978). *Psychometric Theory* (2nd ed.). New York: McGraw-Hill.

Pecora, P., Whittaker J., & Maluccio, A. (1992). *The child welfare challenge.* Hawthorn, NY: Aldine de Gruyter.

Raycraft, J. (1994). The party isn't over: The agency role in the retention of public child welfare caseworkers. *Social Work, 39,* 75-80.

Reagh, R. (1994). Public child welfare professionals: Those who stay. *Journal of Sociology and Social Welfare, 21,* 69-78.

Russell, M., & Hornby, H. (1987). *1987 national study of public child welfare job requirements.* Portland, ME: National Child Welfare Resource Center for Management and Administration.

Social Security Act of 1935, as amended, Amendments of 1994, Title IV-E, Pub. L. 103-432, § 470 *et seq.*

Vinokur-Kaplan, D. (1991). Job satisfaction among social workers in public and voluntary child welfare agencies. *Child Welfare, 70,* 81-91.

Factors Influencing the Retention of Specially Educated Public Child Welfare Workers

Nancy S. Dickinson, PhD
Robin E. Perry, PhD

SUMMARY. Although public child welfare has historically been a major employer of professional social workers, within the last twenty years MSW graduates have shunned public social services for the private sector. Using Title IV-E funds, universities have responded to this shortage by providing financial and educational incentives for graduate social work students to work with the diverse and complex cases in public child welfare. As a result, the numbers of graduate social workers seeking employment in public child welfare have increased, but questions remain about the extent to which professional social workers remain employed in public child welfare agencies beyond their employment payback period. This paper reports the results of one research study on the factors that affect the retention of these master's level child welfare workers. *[Article copies available for a fee from The Haworth Document Delivery Service: 1-800-HAWORTH. E-mail address: <getinfo@haworthpressinc.com> Website: <http://www.HaworthPress.com> © 2002 by The Haworth Press, Inc. All rights reserved.]*

Nancy S. Dickinson is Clinical Professor and Director, Jordan Institute for Families, School of Social Work, University of North Carolina at Chapel Hill.

Robin E. Perry is Assistant Professor, School of Social Work, Florida State University, Tallahassee, FL.

This research was supported by the California Department of Social Services with federal Title IV-E support.

[Haworth co-indexing entry note]: "Factors Influencing the Retention of Specially Educated Public Child Welfare Workers." Dickinson, Nancy S., and Robin E. Perry. Co-published simultaneously in *Journal of Health & Social Policy* (The Haworth Press, Inc.) Vol. 15, No. 3/4, 2002, pp. 89-103; and: *Evaluation Research in Child Welfare: Improving Outcomes Through University-Public Agency Partnerships* (ed: Katharine Briar-Lawson, and Joan Levy Zlotnik) The Haworth Press, Inc., 2002, pp. 89-103. Single or multiple copies of this article are available for a fee from The Haworth Document Delivery Service [1-800-HAWORTH, 9:00 a.m. - 5:00 p.m. (EST). E-mail address: getinfo@haworthpressinc.com].

KEYWORDS. Child welfare workers, retention, burnout, Title IV-E, workplace supports

BACKGROUND

Public child welfare agencies have long been key training and employment settings for professional social workers (Rubin, 1981; Sheehan, 1976; CSWE, 1960; Bureau of Labor Statistics, 1952). Regardless, within the last twenty years, the deprofessionalization of many public sector jobs has made those positions unappealing to professionally educated social workers (Leighninger & Ellett, 1998; Dressel et al., 1988; Groulx, 1983; Getzel, 1983). Specific concern is focused on the limited number of MSWs employed in public child welfare services, since several studies suggest that those child welfare workers with MSWs are more competent and better prepared for the stresses typically encountered in public child welfare services than non-MSWs (Dhooper, Royse, & Wolfe, 1990; Liebermann et al., 1988; Booz-Allen & Hamilton, 1987; University of Southern Maine, 1987). Many of these authors also suggested that states with minimum degree requirements of a BSW or an MSW for public child welfare staff have lower vacancy and turnover rates than states with no such requirements. These studies, however, differ in design rigor and their representative nature.

In addition to understanding how to increase the numbers of qualified professionals in public child welfare, it is important to know those factors that affect their retention. In a recent study of public child welfare workers in Oklahoma, Rosenthal, McDowell, and White (1998) found the following variables to be positively associated with higher retention rates:

1. age when the worker started in public child welfare;
2. time worked in a Department of Human Services agency before beginning work specifically in child welfare services; and
3. possession of a masters degree in a human service area other than social work.

Public child welfare workers who participated in a Title IV-E funded training program did not remain employed longer than those without such training. Other studies have focused on the role of worker age, ethnicity and gender in retention of public social services workers (McNeely 1992; 1989; Jayaratne & Chess, 1984).

Additional studies on retention rates are not multi-dimensional in nature. Within this context, worker turnover rates have been positively associated with budget reductions and fears of layoffs (McNeely, 1992); limited or low monetary and non-monetary benefits (Henry, 1990; Herzberg, 1966); general job dissatisfaction (Mailick, 1991; Oktay, 1992); and the age of the agency and its physical environment or "organizational conditions" (Glisson & Durick, 1988; Weiner, 1991).

Since child protection workers, on average, experience higher levels of stress and role conflict than social workers employed in other settings (Jayaratne & Chess, 1984), stress and burnout may relate to retention. General studies of stress and burnout among social workers have focused on:

1. the importance of social supports within and outside of the work place (Jayaratne, Chess, & Kundel, 1986; Davis-Sacks, Jayarnte, & Chess, 1985);
2. work place financial and non-financial rewards and conditions (Jayaratne & Chess, 1984);
3. caseload size and demands (Maslach & Jackson, 1984); and
4. specific job functions and activities of child welfare workers (Vinokur-Kaplan & Hartman, 1986).

A number of variables have been examined for their influence on job satisfaction, which may also relate to retention. Vinokur-Kaplan et al. (1994) cite studies (McNeely, 1989; O'Toole, 1973) that equate low levels of job satisfaction with a decrease in the health, mental health, job effectiveness, and social functioning of workers. Other authors examine the importance of specific job factors on job satisfaction, including workload, work place comfort and safety, job challenges (and feelings of accomplishment), financial awards, promotional opportunities, social supports, role conflict and role ambiguity (Rauktis & Koeske, 1994; Tracy et al., 1992; Koeske & Koeske, 1989; Vinokur-Kaplan, 1991; Glisson & Durick, 1988; Jayaratne & Chess, 1982-83). Samantrai (1992) adds that job satisfaction is also influenced by the status that is afforded someone with an MSW degree and their public image and liability. Given the multitude of potential influences considered in the literature, there is a need for studies that consider a range of variables in models used to predict worker retention in public child welfare.

Popular support in California for increasing the numbers of MSWs in public child welfare led to the creation of the California Social Work Education Center (CalSWEC) in 1990 through the collaborative efforts of the deans and directors of California graduate schools of social work and the County Welfare Directors Association (which represents 58 county departments of social Services). In 1992, through a contract with the California Department of Social Services using federal Title IV-E training funds, CalSWEC began a Child Welfare Stipend Program that provides financial support for graduate students who pursue careers in public child welfare. Stipended students participate in a specialized curriculum based on the knowledge, skills and attitudes which are needed for child welfare practice. Upon graduation, the students are required to work one year in a public child welfare agency for each year of funding they received.

This study presents preliminary findings from a longitudinal study of CalSWEC's success in increasing the number of MSW graduates employed in public child welfare positions. In particular, this paper focuses on those Title IV-E stipended participants who have completed their contractual obligation to work in a public child welfare agency. The graduates who remain are compared to those who left public child welfare employment. Efforts are made to identify those factors most likely to influence the retention of specially trained social workers in public child welfare positions.

METHOD

The researchers mailed a self-administered survey instrument to every social worker who received Title IV-E funding from CalSWEC during graduate school. The survey was mailed to these social workers between three and six months following the completion of their contractual obligation to work in a county public child welfare agency (or employment payback). As of June 1999, a total of 368 former CalSWEC participants were surveyed.

The survey instrument consists of three sections. The first section asks questions related to work experiences in public child welfare, including job roles and responsibilities, the size and demands of each subject's caseload, the breakdown of their caseload by ethnicity, and the perceived nature and level of supervisory and social supports respondents typically relied upon while employed in child welfare services. Additional questions attempt to determine the likelihood that each respondent will seek alternative employment in the near future and the potential reasons for their decision to leave public child welfare employment. While the researchers developed many of these questions, several were adapted from other studies (Vinokur-Kaplan et al., 1994; Himle, Jayarante & Thyness, 1989; House, 1981; House & Wells, 1978).

Questions in the instrument's second section address each subject's perceptions of work conditions, including the extent to which each respondent feels "burned out" as a child welfare worker. To help facilitate this line of inquiry, the Maslach Burnout Inventory (MBI) is integrated into the questionnaire. A copyrighted instrument, the MBI has been modified for human service professionals and consists of subscales measuring three dimensions of the "burnout syndrome": emotional exhaustion, depersonalization, and lack of personal accomplishment. Each subscale has demonstrated internal reliability as well as convergent and discriminant validity when used with a variety of service professionals. Normative sample scores of "social service workers" (which include social workers and child protection workers) detailed by Maslach and Jackson (1986) are used as a guide for interpreting the level of burnout experienced by respondents in this study.

In addition to the MBI, the second section includes questions adapted from other studies (Tracy et al., 1992; Jayaratne, Chess, & Kunkel, 1986) on the level of stress associated with specific duties or situations in child welfare services and measure the level of satisfaction each respondent has with a variety of employment related experiences. Finally, five questions (taken from Ellett et al., 1996) elicit each respondent's views on the quality and efficacy of their work in child welfare.

The third section of the questionnaire relates to personal or socio-demographic variables. These include the age, sex, ethnicity, relationship status, religious affiliation, political and ideological affiliations, socio-economic status while growing up and time spent in a variety of non-work activities each week.

FINDINGS

Determining the Retention Rate of Title IV-E Stipended MSWs

As of June 1999, 368 Title IV-E stipended CalSWEC participants–who completed their employment payback–had been surveyed. As noted earlier, each potential respondent was typically surveyed between three and six months following the completion of his or her employment payback.

Of these 368 potential study subjects, 78.0% (n = 287) remained employed in public child welfare (either in the agency where they completed their employment payback or at another county child welfare agency). A total of 81 (22.0%) study subjects were no longer working in the public child welfare agency where they completed their employment payback. Of these subjects, 27 were employed in a setting other than a public child welfare agency. The remaining 54 subjects could not be located. Given that 12 of the 287 subjects still in public child welfare were employed in a different public child welfare agency, it is possible that a small proportion of those who could not be located were employed in another county child welfare agency, thus under-estimating the actual retention rate of Title IV-E stipended social workers in public child welfare.

Of the 368 social workers surveyed, 63.9% (n = 235) completed the survey instrument. The moderate response rate occurred because of a large number of incorrect mailing addresses. These 235 respondents are the subjects of this paper.

Among those subjects who responded to the survey (n = 235), 88.5% (n = 208) were still employed in a public child welfare agency. This retention rate is larger than that observed when the entire population of potential respondents is considered. A chi-square test (between the distribution of all potential cases according to whether they responded to the survey by their current employ-ment status) revealed that those still employed in public child welfare are sig-nificantly over-represented among those who responded to the survey (χ^2 = 41.93, df = 1, p < .0001). Any findings presented henceforth are qualified by this observation.

Group Comparisons Using Survey Data

A total of 65 study subjects of the 235 social workers who responded to the survey were employed at that time in a public child welfare agency but indi-cated that they planned (or reported a likelihood within the next year) to leave public child welfare employment. When these subjects are combined with those respondents who had already left public child welfare, 39.1% (n = 92) of survey respondents had left or planned to leave public child welfare and 60.9% (n = 143) remained and reportedly intended to remain in public child welfare over the next year. In this section, survey responses of those who left or in-tended to leave public child welfare are compared with the responses of those who remained and intended to remain in public child welfare.

A series of bi-variate analyses (using t-tests and chi-square tests where ap-plicable) was conducted with a multitude of variables (interval and categori-cal) where respondents' forecasted retention status (did they stay and did they intend to stay in public child welfare or not) served as the grouping variable. The unbalanced nature of the principal grouping variable may affect the accu-racy of test statistics generated, as these statistics will typically have large con-fidence intervals. Any assumption violations call into question the accuracy of probability values generated for hypotheses testing. To address these con-cerns, the researchers tested the normality of each variable distribution for each forecasted retention group using the Lilliefors test. Further, the Levene's test was used to test whether variances were equal. Should the assumption of normality be violated, the researchers used nonparametric procedures (the Wilcoxon Rank Sum W test with interval level variables) to test for differences between groups. If normality assumptions were met and variances were not equal, separate variance–as opposed to pooled variance–estimates were used in t-tests. Where assumptions of normality and equal variances were violated, the researchers discarded the analyses results.

Job Characteristics

Several questions solicited information about a respondent's:

1. time spent in specific service areas (emergency response, court services, family maintenance, family reunification, adoptions, foster care, or fam-ily preservation);
2. salary;

3. work hours, caseload size and type; and
4. time spent doing administrative versus service activities.

When number of months spent in different service areas is considered, no significant differences are observed between both retention groups. This conflicts with preliminary findings on these data (Dickinson & Perry, 1998) where those who stay in public child welfare reported a significantly higher mean number of months' work in adoptions and permanency planning than those who left or plan to leave public child welfare.

Those who left or plan to leave public child welfare–on average–have an annual salary that was $2,778 less than those who plan to stay in public child welfare ($38,986 compared to $41,764, respectively). This difference is statistically significant (t = -3.24, df = 221, p = .001). In addition, those who have stayed in public child welfare report a statistically higher (t = -1.98, df = 222, p = .049) mean percentage of African Americans on their caseload (μ = 28.24%, S.D. = 24.55) than those who left or plan to leave public child welfare (μ = 21.66%, S.D. = 23.95).

No significant differences were observed between groups in terms of the percentage of time they spend in various administrative and service related responsibilities apart from time spent doing "other" tasks. Here, those who are staying in public child welfare report a significantly lower mean percentage of their workweek (μ = 3.04%) dedicated to "other" tasks than is reported by those who have left or plan to leave public child welfare (μ = 7.83%; t = 2.61, df = 117.29, p = .01). When the nature of these "other" tasks is examined it appears those who have left or plan to leave public child welfare are more likely to be involved in court related tasks (testifying, writing reports and meeting with lawyers).

Although no significant differences were observed between groups in terms of the percentage of respondents who felt their caseload was either "too low" or "about right" versus "too high," those workers who planned on staying in public child welfare carried an average caseload that was significantly higher (μ = 39.24) than that observed among workers who left or planned to leave public child welfare (μ = 34.35; t = -2.23, df = 199.55, p = .027). This finding suggests that the size of a caseload alone is not a reliable predictor of whether or not a worker will leave public child welfare. Although no information is available regarding the demands that individual cases had on individual workers, those who plan to remain in public child welfare appear to be able to manage larger caseloads across a variety of service areas and departments and are no more likely to perceive their caseloads as being "too high" than those who have left or plan to leave public child welfare.

Social Supports Within and Outside of the Agency

The researchers asked several questions about the extent to which respondents felt they received various forms of support from their "immediate supervisor," "other people at work," "friends and relatives," and their "spouse or partner."

No differences were observed between groups in terms of the level or kind of reported support received from friends and family and spouses or partners. These groups differed, however, in the mean level of reported support received from work peers and supervisors. Here, those remaining in public child welfare reported higher levels of support from work peers when ". . . things get tough at work" ($t = -2.00$, df = 232, p = . 046) and in terms of listening ". . . to work related problems" ($t = -2.68$, df = 231, p = .008) and helping respondents get their ". . . job done" ($t = -2.24$, df = 232, p = .026) than those who have left who plan to leave public child welfare.

In addition, significant differences were reported in the levels of support received from respondents' supervisors. Those respondents remaining in public child welfare rated their supervisors at a significantly higher level in terms of: (1) willingness to listen to respondent's work related problems ($t = -3.34$, df = 232, p = .001); (2) extent to which supervisors can be relied on "when things get tough at work" ($t = -3.77$, df = 168.01, p < .001); and (3) helping respondents in getting their job done ($t = -3.99$, df = 167.98, p < .001).

Significant differences were observed between the study groups in terms of their views on the skills and characteristics of their supervisors. Those respondents remaining in public child welfare rated their supervisors as:

1. more competent in doing their job ($t = -3.14$, df = 156.13, p = .002);
2. more concerned with their subordinates' welfare ($t = -3.91$, df = 231, p < .001);
3. more likely to show approval to respondents when they have done a good job ($t = -3.40$, df = 232, p = .001);
4. more likely to help respondents complete difficult tasks ($t = -3.36$, df = 232, p = .001); and
5. more likely to be "warm and friendly" when the respondent is having "problems" ($t = -3.46$, df = 232, p = .001).

Job Satisfaction

Respondents were asked to rate (on a five-point Likert-type scale) the extent to which they were satisfied with twenty-two practice and work environment conditions. Those remaining in public child welfare experienced significantly higher levels of satisfaction on the job with respect to nine of these conditions:

1. "support and recognition from my supervisor" ($t = -2.61$, df = 167.8);

2. "opportunities for personal growth and development" (t = −2.42, df = 231, p = .016);
3. "opportunities for promotion" (t = −2.06, df = 231, p = .041);
4. "opportunities for improving knowledge and skills" (t = −2.52, df = 231, p = .013);
5. "personal feelings of accomplishment" on the job (t = −3.01, df = 161.8, p = .003);
6. "recognition from other professionals" (t = −2.12, df = 231, p = .035);
7. "the authority to make professional decisions" (t = −3.44, df = 230, p = .001);
8. opportunities to "... make a difference in a client's life" (t = −2.08, df = 174.02, p = .039); and
9. the extent to which they were globally satisfied with their job (t = −5.92, df = 155.19, p < .001).

In response to questions assessing their beliefs about their practice and efficacy as child welfare workers, those remaining in public child welfare reported feeling a significantly higher level of influence in positively affecting their clients (t = −2.93, df = 230, p = .004).

Demographic Differences

No significant differences (using chi-square tests) occur in the distribution of those who remained versus left public child welfare according to their gender or race/ethnicity (white/non-white), or the socio-demographic status (low, middle or upper) of respondents' families during their youth. Further, there are no significant differences between retention groups in terms of the mean age of respondents (μ = 36.49 years for those who remained and μ = 36.34 years for those who left).

Reasons for Leaving

Respondents who left or were likely to leave public child welfare (n = 92) were asked to rate on a five-point Likert-type scale the level of importance for which nine statements influenced their decision to leave public child welfare. Among these nine statements, the four most important reasons include:

1. feeling "burned out" or over stressed (μ = 4.05, S.D. = 1.09);
2. dissatisfaction with current job/work environment (μ = 3.85, S.D. = 1.21);
3. changes in career goals (μ = 3.21, S.D. = 1.26); and
4. the availability of other jobs (μ = 3.18, S.D. = 1.27).

Given the prominence that feeling "burned out" or over stressed had upon workers' desire to leave public child welfare, it seems important to examine the dimensions, prevalence and influence of these variables with all study subjects.

Burnout and Stress

The level of experienced "burnout" or job stress was principally measured using the three subscales of the Maslach Burnout Inventory that measure emotional exhaustion, depersonalization, and lack of personal accomplishment experienced on the job. Study subjects did not differ in the level of personal accomplishment and sense of depersonalization experienced on the job. Although the mean level of personal accomplishment was higher for those who stayed (μ = 36.56) than those who left public child welfare (μ = 35.27), these differences are not statistically significant and suggest that both groups–on average–experience similar levels of personal accomplishment that are not associated with high levels of burnout. Likewise, both groups–on average–experience the same level of depersonalization (μ = 7.82 and μ = 8.48 for those who stayed versus left public child welfare, respectively) which are not associated with high levels of burnout.

There are significant differences, however, in the mean levels of emotional exhaustion experienced by both groups of study subjects (t = 4.75, df = 231, p < .001). Those who left or were likely to leave public child welfare experienced mean levels of emotional exhaustion (μ = 29.98) associated with high levels of burnout (see Maslach and Jackson, 1986). The mean level of emotional exhaustion (μ = 23.54) experienced by those who remained in public child welfare is associated with average levels of burnout. These findings are consistent with Brett and Yadama's (1996) study (as cited in Rosenthal et al., 1998) of 177 child protection workers in Missouri where emotional exhaustion had a significant effect on job exit.

As noted earlier, in addition to the Maslach Burnout Inventory, the researchers asked a series of other questions regarding the stress that specific duties or situations affiliated with child welfare services might cause for each respondent. Interestingly, both groups of study subjects were similar in the mean levels of stress they experienced with respect to all situations or duties except one. Those who left or were likely to leave public child welfare report higher levels of stress associated with "needing to work overtime" than those who remained and planned to stay in public child welfare (t = 2.37, df = 229, p = .019). However, no significant differences are observed between groups in terms of the average hours worked each week (t = 1.04, df = 146.76, p = .295), which is 43.67 hours (S.D. = 6.33) and 42.87 hours (S.D. = 4.45) for those who left or planned to leave and those who planned to remain in public child welfare, respectively.

Multiple Logistic Regression Model

Given the significant differences between subject groups across a number of variables (using a series of bi-variate analyses), multiple logistic regression procedures were employed to develop a more parsimonious model of variable effects upon worker retention. The dependent variable is the respondents' status regarding whether or not they stayed and planned to stay in public child welfare at the time they were surveyed (n = 235). Independent variables included all those variables for which a significant difference in their distribution existed (using a series of simple bi-variate analyses) between these two groups of Title IV-E stipended MSW graduates, as presented earlier.

Table 1 details results using a forward logistic regression model. These findings suggest that among the large number of variables shown to have a significant association with retention rates using bi-variate analyses, only five variables significantly influence the likelihood that a specially educated Title IV-E stipended MSW graduate will remain employed in public child welfare beyond their employment payback requirement. Here, workers' salaries and the level of social supports received from co-workers and their supervisors positively influence the retention rate of public child welfare workers. With respect to supervisory support, the greater the extent to which workers perceived their supervisor as being very concerned about their welfare, the greater the likelihood respondents would remain in public child welfare. Given the many ways by which a supervisor can show concern for worker's welfare, it is thought that this variable serves as a latent variable for the seven additional items associated with specific supervisory supports that demonstrated a significant influence upon retention rates when bi-variate analyses were conducted. In addition, findings in Table 1 suggest that as the level of emotional exhaustion and the percentage of time spent doing "other" tasks (court related activities) increase, there is a significant decrease in the retention of public child welfare workers.

CONCLUSION

Public child welfare services reach families with complex needs and children in imminent danger. They deserve the highest level of professional expertise. Title IV-E funded educational and financial incentives have increased the numbers of graduate social workers seeking employment in public child welfare, but these incentives are not sufficient for retaining professional social workers in public child welfare agencies beyond their employment payback period. This study adds to the growing body of research on the factors that affect the retention of these workers.

TABLE 1. Forward Stepwise Logistic Regression of Independent Variables on the Likelihood that Respondents Stayed and Intended to Stay in Public Child Welfare After Completing Their Employment Payback (n = 208)*

Dependent variable = whether or not respondents stayed and intended to stay in public child welfare.			
Independent Variables	β (sig. β)	Exp (β)	R
Level of emotional exhaustion as measured by the Maslach Burnout Inventory	−.0446 (p = .0076)	.9564	−.1363
Salary of respondent	.000088 (p = .0022)	1.0001	.1634
Percentage of work week spent doing "other" tasks	−.0333 (p = .0173)	.9673	−.1154
The extent to which "other people at work" listen to the respondents about work-related problems	.5935 (p = .0168)	1.8103	.1163
Level to which supervisor is very concerned about the welfare of workers under him/her	.6167 (p = .0056)	1.8529	.1435
Constant $β_0$	−5.839		

* Using listwise deletion procedures, n = 27 cases were excluded from the final model. A chi-square test (χ^2 = .405, p = .524) suggests that the distribution of cases included versus excluded from the model in Table 1 is independent of the distribution of cases according to their status as staying versus left/leaving public child welfare. Therefore, cases excluded from the final model (in Table 1) are randomly distributed with respect to the dependent variable.

The findings show that 78% of one group of 368 California MSWs who received Title IV-E funded stipends and educational support remained employed in public child welfare three to six months after their employment payback requirement ended. While this rate may underestimate the true retention rate of specially trained MSWs, it is also possible that the rate is no different from–or even less than–the retention rate of child welfare staff with other degrees, since there was no control group of MSW graduates who did not receive special funding or educational curricula. Future studies of this nature should have such a control group.

In spite of these limitations, the results of a survey of the IV-E funded MSW graduates show some informative differences between the graduates who remained in public child welfare positions and those who left or intended to leave. The social workers who remained in public child welfare employment were less emotionally exhausted, earned higher salaries, spent less time on court related tasks and reported receiving more support from work peers and supervisors than social workers who left or planned to leave public child welfare jobs. Worker retention in this study was not affected by age, race, or job service area.

Worker burnout was the number one reason for leaving given by subjects who had left or were likely to leave public child welfare employment. Burnout may have contributed to dissatisfaction with their jobs and led subsequently to changes in their career goals and to the awareness of the availability of other jobs–other reasons respondents listed for leaving public child welfare employment.

In this study, emotional exhaustion was the type of burnout that distinguished the leavers from those workers who remained on their jobs. While both groups experienced similar levels of personal accomplishment, that sense of efficacy was not enough to promote retention. Rather, the ability to form relationships with work peers where work-related problems were discussed and to rely on supervisors for support seemed to buffer those who remained on the job from the difficulties and isolation–and exhaustion–of public child welfare work.

REFERENCES

Booz-Allen and Hamilton, Inc. (1987). *The Maryland social work service job analysis and personnel qualifications study.*

Bureau of Labor Statistics. (1952). *Social workers in 1950.* New York: American Association of Social Workers.

Council on Social Work Education. (1960). *Statistics on social work education: November 1, 1960 and Academic Year 1959-60.* New York: Council on Social Work Education.

Davis-Sacks, M., Jayaratne, S., & Chess, W. (1985). A comparison of the effects of social support on the incidence of burnout. *Social Work, 30* (3), 240-244.

Dhooper, S., Royse, D., & Wolfe, L. (1990). Does social work education make a difference? *Social Work, 35* (1), 57-61.

Dickinson, N., & Perry, R. (1998). *Do M.S.W. graduates stay in public child welfare?* Paper presented at the 38th Annual National Association for Welfare Research and Statistics Conference. Chicago, IL, August 4.

Dressel, P., Waters, M., Sweat, M., Clayton, O., & Chandler-Clayton, A. (1988). Deprofessionalization, proletarianization, and social welfare work. *Journal of Sociology and Social Welfare, 15* (2), 113-131.

Ellett, C. D., Ellett, A. J., Kelley, B. L., & Naoble, D. N. (1996). *A statewide study of child welfare personnel needs: Who stays? Who leaves? Who cares?* Paper presented at the 42nd annual program meeting of the Council on Social Work Education, Washington DC.

Getzel, G. S. (1983). Speculations on the crisis in social work recruitment: Some modest proposals. *Social Work, 28* (3), 235-237.

Glisson, C., & Durick, M. (1988). Predictors of job satisfaction and organizational committment in human service organizations. *Administrative Science Quarterly, 33* (1), 61-81.

Groulx, L. (1983). Deprofessionalization of social services: Demands of democracy or pretensions to a new power? *International Social Work, 26* (3), 38-44.

Henry, S. (1990). Non-salary retention incentives for social workers in public mental health. *Administration in Social Work, 14* (3), 1-15.

Herzberg, F. (1966). *Work and the nature of man.* Cleveland: World Publishing Company.

Himle, D., Jayaratne, S., & Thyness, P. (1989). The buffering effects of four types of supervisory support on work stress. *Administration in Social Work, 13* (1), 19-33.

House, J. S. (1981). *Work stress and social support.* Menlo Park, CA: Addison-Wesley Publishing Company.

House, J. S., & Wells, J. A. (1978). Occupational stress, social support, and health. In A. McLean, G. Black and M. Colligan (Eds.), *Reducing occupational stress: Proceedings of a conference.* DHEW (NIOSH) Publication 78-140: 8-29.

Jayaratne, S., Chess, W. A., & Kunkel, D. A. (1986). Burnout: Its impact on child welfare workers and their spouses. *Social Work, 31* (1), 53-60.

Jayaratne, S., & Chess, W. A. (1984). Job satisfaction, burnout, and turnover: A national study. *Social Work, 29* (5), 448-453.

Jayaratne, S., & Chess, W. A. (1982-83). Some correlates of job satisfaction among social workers. *The Journal of Applied Social Sciences, 7* (1), 1-17.

Koeske, G. & Koeske, R. D. (1989) Work load and burnout: Can social support and perceived accomplishment help? *Social Work,* May, 243-248.

Leighninger, L. & Ellett, A. J. (1998). *De-professionalization in child welfare: Historical analysis and implications for social work education.* Paper presented at the APM of the Council on Social Work Education, March 7, 1998.

Liebermann, A., Hornby, H., & Russell, M. (1988). Analyzing the educational backgrounds and work experiences of child welfare personnel: A national study. *Social Work, 33* (6), 485-489.

Mailick, M. D. (1991). Recruitment and retention of MSW graduates. *Social Work in Health Care, 16* (2), 1-4.

Maslach, C., & Jackson, S. E. (1986). *Maslach Burnout Inventory: Manual.* Palo Alto, CA: Consulting Psychologists Press, Inc.

Maslach, C., & Jackson, S. E. (1984). Patterns of burnout among a national sample of public contact workers. *Journal of Health and Human Resources Administration, 7,* 189-212.

McNeely, R. L. (1992). Job satisfaction in the public social services: Perspectives on structure, situational factors, gender and ethnicity. In Y. Hasenfeld (Ed.), *Human services as complex organizations.* Beverly Hills, CA: Sage Publications.

McNeely, R. L. (1989). Gender, job satisfaction, earning and other characteristics of human service workers during and after midlife. *Administration in Social Work, 13* (2), 99-116.

Oktay, J. S. (1992). Burnout in hospital social workers who work with AIDS patients. *Social Work, 37* (5), 432-439.

O'Toole, J. (Ed.). (1973). *Work in America: Report of a special task force to the Secretary of Health, Education and Welfare.* Cambridge, MA: MIT Press.

Rauktis, M., & Koeske, G. (1994). Maintaining social worker morale: When supportive supervision is not enough. *Administration in Social Work, 18* (1), 3-60.

Rosenthal, J. A., McDowell, E. C., & White, T. L. (1998). *Retention of child welfare workers in Oklahoma.* University of Oklahoma School of Social Work.

Rubin, A. (1981). *Statistics on social work education in the United States: 1980.* New York: Council on Social Work Education.

Samantrai, K. (1992). Factors in the decision to leave: Retaining social workers with MSWs in public child welfare. *Social Work, 37* (5), 454-458.

Sheehan, J. C. (1976). *Statistics on social work education: 1975.* New York: Council on Social Work Education.

Tracy, E. M., Bean, N., Gwatkin, S., & Hill, B. (1992). Family preservation workers: Sources of job satisfaction and job stress. *Research on Social Work Practice, 2* (4), 465-478.

University of Southern Maine. (1987). *Professional social work practice in public child welfare: An agenda for action.* National Child Welfare Resource Center for Management Administration, Portland, ME: Author.

Vinokur-Kaplan, D. (1991). Job satisfaction among social workers in public and voluntary child welfare agencies. *Child Welfare, 70* (1), 81-91.

Vinokur-Kaplan, D., & Hartman, A. (1986). A national profile of child welfare workers and supervisors. *Child Welfare, 65* (4), 323-335.

Vinokur-Kaplan, D., Jayaratne, S., & Chess, W. A. (1994). Job satisfaction and retention of social workers in public agencies, non-profit agencies, and private practice: The impact of workplace conditions and motivators. *Administration in Social Work, 18* (3), 93-121.

Weiner, M. E. (1991). Motivating employees to achieve. In R. E. Edwards et al. (Eds.), *Skills for effective human services management.* Silver Spring, MD: NASW.

Tracking Process and Outcome Results of BSW Students' Preparation for Public Child Welfare Practice: Lessons Learned

J. Karen Brown, PhD
Nancy Feyl Chavkin, PhD
Vevelyn Peterson, LMSW

SUMMARY. A Texas university/agency partnership program to prepare social work students for public child welfare conducted an exploratory study of the process and outcome results of the program's efforts from 1989-99 and offers recommendations to other university/agency programs. The evaluation plan was multi-faceted, and the evaluation included both process and outcome components from the perspectives of each stakeholder–the agency, the university, the students, the clients, and the taxpayers. The paper concludes with recommendations for the future. The partnership acknowledges that these evaluation results have limitations and are not generalizable beyond this specific partnership. The lessons learned in this university/agency partnership are first steps in developing better partnerships to prepare students for public child welfare practice. *[Article copies available for a fee from The Haworth Document Delivery Service: 1-800-HAWORTH. E-mail address: <getinfo@haworthpressinc.com> Website: <http://www.HaworthPress.com> © 2002 by The Haworth Press, Inc. All rights reserved.]*

J. Karen Brown, Nancy Feyl Chavkin, and Vevelyn Peterson are all affiliated with the Center for Children and Families at Southwest Texas State University, 601 University Drive, San Marcos, TX 78666.

[Haworth co-indexing entry note]: "Tracking Process and Outcome Results of BSW Students' Preparation for Public Child Welfare Practice: Lessons Learned." Brown, J. Karen , Nancy Feyl Chavkin, and Vevelyn Peterson. Co-published simultaneously in *Journal of Health & Social Policy* (The Haworth Press, Inc.) Vol. 15, No. 3/4, 2002, pp. 105-116; and: *Evaluation Research in Child Welfare: Improving Outcomes Through University-Public Agency Partnerships* (ed: Katharine Briar-Lawson, and Joan Levy Zlotnik) The Haworth Press, Inc., 2002, pp. 105-116. Single or multiple copies of this article are available for a fee from The Haworth Document Delivery Service [1-800-HAWORTH, 9:00 a.m. - 5:00 p.m. (EST). E-mail address: getinfo@haworthpressinc.com].

KEYWORDS. Child welfare, partnership, training, Title IV-E, social work, evaluation, outcomes

The evidence is incontrovertible; there is a tremendous need for professionally prepared social workers in public child welfare. Child abuse rates are at all time high and worker turnover is escalating. In the state of Texas most new child welfare workers stay fewer than 21 months on the job, and in some regions workers do not come back after the first day on the job (Hollandsworth, 1998). Child welfare practice has become more challenging than ever before in American history (Leighninger and Ellett, 1998), and the challenges ahead in the new millennium promise to become even more complex. To add to this crisis, national and state studies on social work career choices indicate that fewer than 28% of the workers entering the child welfare field have a professional social work education (Alperin, 1998; Baer & McLean, 1994; Lieberman, Hornby, & Russell, 1988; Pecora, Briar, & Zlotnik, 1989; Rome, 1994). This paper briefly

1. describes a Texas university/agency partnership program to prepare social work students for public child welfare,
2. reports on an exploratory study of the process and outcome results of the program's efforts, and
3. offers recommendations to other university/agency programs.

Like many social education programs (Zlotnik, 1997), the partnership received assistance from both Title IV-B (426) and Title IV-E funds for the ten-year period from 1989-1999.

Because the partnership effort has been evolutionary, the evaluation plan was multi-faceted, and evaluation included both process and outcome components from the perspectives of three primary stakeholders–the agency, the university, and the students. After describing the partnership efforts, part two of the paper reports on the process evaluation, and part three describes the outcome evaluation thus far. The paper concludes with recommendations for the future. The partnership acknowledges that these evaluation results have limitations and are not generalizable beyond this specific partnership. The purpose in reporting the exploratory study of the process and outcome evaluation data to date is to help other programs develop better evaluation processes to understand more about the complex nature of university/agency partnerships for preparing students for public child welfare. The lessons learned in this university/agency partnership are first-steps in developing better partnerships to prepare students for public child welfare practice.

DESCRIPTION OF THE UNIVERSITY/AGENCY PARTNERSHIP

The first 426 grant built on a long-term, positive relationship between the University and the local Child Protective Service (CPS) agency. The university developed a Child Welfare Sequence (see Figure 1) that included elective coursework in child welfare, minorities, and alcohol and drugs, and a summer Intensive Spanish Language Institute for social work students. The focus of the partnership project was to recruit BSW graduates to address the broad needs of the child welfare population. Scholarships were awarded to any BSW major who was interested in child welfare. The agency partners were supportive but not actively involved in the curriculum aspects of the program.

The next grants continued the Child Welfare Sequence and had two additional components: more emphasis on the recruitment of minority students and a focus on the hiring needs of the public child welfare agency. The partners expanded to include active participation by not only the Institute of Social Work and the Department of Modern Language but also the personnel recruiter from the state department of public child welfare, the training director for the two nearby child welfare regions, and key administrators of both the state and regional offices. Students were strongly encouraged and recruited to accept employment at CPS.

The following year, the partnership agreed to focus the program on students in the final college semester who were placed in full-time internships with CPS. Student interns participated in the Basic Job Skills Training (BJST) as part of their internship and were hired immediately following the internship. Because the students had passed the BJST during the internship, they were ready to go to work in public child welfare. The agency partners demonstrated increased commitment to the project because these interns were clearly in line to become their employees. For the first time, students signed a contract requiring them to go to work for TDPRS or repay their scholarship. The partners expanded to include the new BSW programs.

With the advent of Title IV-E funding, the partnership was able to further develop curriculum and hire additional faculty and a grant secretary. Faculty were hired to teach in the Child Welfare Sequence, and we were able to offer more classes and smaller classes related to child welfare. The curriculum development component focused on developing modules and class presentations related to the generalist curriculum (practice, policy, and field courses were targeted). An innovative Spanish Language videotape and computer-assisted instruction program was developed specifically for social workers. Faculty participated in in-service education activities at state and national meetings. Additional curriculum units were developed in the areas of child welfare and grandparents, alcoholism, and respite care. In addition to the scholarships for full-time internships, students competed for six mini-scholarships for poster

FIGURE 1. Child Welfare Sequence

Elective Course

Social Work 4315: Child Welfare Services
(This elective course covers the following topics: historical context of child welfare services, family dynamics, child development, cultural diversity issues, child maltreatment, types and scope of child welfare services, future directions and priorities in child welfare services.)

Plus

One Additional Elective Course

(Emphasizing in more depth diversity issues and family dynamics, particularly the relation-ship between addiction and family dynamics.)

Social Work 4310: Social Services with Minorities

Or

Social Work 3312: Alcohol and Drugs

Plus

The Intensive Spanish Language Institute for Social Workers
(This is an intensive summer-long study of primarily conversational Spanish using social work vocabulary. Students enroll the summer prior to their internship.)

Plus

---

600 Hours of Field Practicum at Child Protective Service Agency
(This is a block placement during the student's final semester of social work education. The students complete a modified version of the agency's Basic Skill Development class and complete all requirements to begin employment upon graduation.)

---

presentations and videos of child welfare related topics. The program held an Invitational Roundtable with other social work faculty and representatives of CPS to discuss developing more partnerships across the state.

As the partnership progressed, the number of students receiving stipends increased. At the request of CPS, we developed a second training unit for social work students. The title of the BJST Training was changed to Basic Skill Development (BSD) to reflect the increased emphasis on continuous skill development. Because the number of partners increased, the frequency of meeting and talking about our goals also increased.

Today, the partnership is graduating approximately 30 students per year, and most are offered full-time positions in CPS upon graduation. A total of 149 students have completed the Child Welfare Sequence. We are collecting and analyzing both process and outcome data, and meeting on a monthly basis with all the partners. The agency personnel are attending and presenting at national and state conferences with faculty, and the university has hired some agency employees.

PROCESS EVALUATION

Process evaluation has been critical to this partnership project because of the complex nature of the relationships involved. The process evaluation reports on benefits and problems from each stakeholder's perspective. Understanding the stakeholders and developing a true university-agency partnership is the first step in conducting an evaluation. If this foundation is not strong, the other steps in data collection will likely either fall by the wayside or not be truly representative of what is happening with the social work graduates.

Like most partnerships, this partnership has faced many challenges, some with more success than others. For example, the first time faculty recommended students for stipends there was an agonizing faculty meeting which focused on which students were most deserving and which were most committed to child welfare practice and how to determine both "deserving" and "committed to child welfare practice." As a result, about half the scholarships went to students with demonstrated financial need and demonstrated commitment to child welfare practice and half to students without financial need but demonstrated commitment to the field. Another time, the faculty felt manipulated by a student who received a stipend and then changed majors. This was the direct result of not having a written contract with the student. Other students wrote beautiful essays about their commitment, completed an internship, and then choose to work in a proprietary agency rather than CPS. Most of these early problems have been addressed as we learned from our mistakes and took action, such as developing guidelines for student selection and requiring formal written contracts with all stipend recipients. The wording of the contract between the student, the university, and the agency has also undergone changes on several occasions. Each time, the revised contract has better reflected the realities of the partnership process.

Staff changes in CPS on the local, regional and state level have been tremendous since the partnership began ten years ago. These staff changes have resulted in the transfer of key contacts to a new division and the evaporation of well-developed relationships. Another time, the state initiated hiring freezes prohibiting local and regional personnel from hiring our social work graduates as planned. We quickly learned to be flexible and adapt. We became more conscientious about writing minutes of all meetings and getting all agreements in writing.

A number of personnel changes have also occurred at the university. We have had new faculty, new administrators, and new accounting procedures. With each change, we had to explain the importance of our partnership and work through a myriad of paperwork to make sure that we were clear about who was paying for what. The very term " stipend" has been through at least two other cycles–once it was " scholarship" and other times it has been "stipend" or "subsistence pay." The university's accounting procedures are sometimes different than either the federal guidelines or the state procedures. The budget year runs on different cycles than the academic year. We have learned to be patient and to be creative in seeking solutions with our colleagues.

The partnership has resulted in many benefits for the regional child welfare agency. CPS is particularly pleased to be able to hire employees who possess an excellent foundation in child welfare and who are motivated to continue their professional development. They draw upon an annual pool of qualified BSW level social workers who are immediately available for employment. These workers have the skills and knowledge of generalist social work practitioners and specialized knowledge in child welfare, social services to minorities, and drug and alcohol dependence. Since the Department of Social Work actively recruits minority students, many of these new workers are bilingual and those that are not will have had intensive training in Spanish.

BSW graduates are individuals who have established a commitment to social work during their four-year, rigorous academic program. In contrast to persons coming out of other academic programs, BSW graduates make better employees in social work positions (Lieberman, Hornby, & Russell, 1988; Dhooper, Royse, & Wolfe, 1990). In addition the graduates completing the Child Welfare Sequence (see Figure 1) at the university are already oriented to the agency as a result of completing the 600-hour public child welfare internship. In the internship, CPS supervisors have had the opportunity to evaluate the job competency of the prospective worker before a hiring decision was made, eliminating some of the risk associated with the investment of training dollars in new workers.

The Child Welfare Sequence has expanded the "generalist" approach required of BSW programs by the Council on Social Work Education (CSWE) to include extensive content on child welfare, social work with minorities, drug and alcohol dependence, and Spanish language training. The final stage in the sequence is the 600-hour public child welfare internship, which requires the full-time participation of the student. This Child Welfare Sequence has been a model for other programs and includes up-to-date information about family preservation, permanency planning, and adoption. The project has allowed for more classes and smaller classes in the Child Welfare Sequence and in the BSW major courses.

New faculty and current faculty have developed special units on child welfare which have been infused into existing BSW generalist courses and allow for all of our BSW graduates to have background information about working in child welfare. Faculty have been provided opportunities for further education and for sharing their ideas about improving child welfare with local, state, and national groups at conferences and meetings. Faculty report that they benefit from being involved with this partnership because it gives them close ties and easy access to what is happening in public sector social work.

Social work students clearly benefited from the financial support provided during their internships. Financial support enabled students to devote their full energy to learning without seeking part-time employment or encouraging additional debt. The established commitment between the child welfare internship and post graduation employment has lessened student's anxiety about entering the job market and allowed them to focus their energy on learning throughout the semester.

BSW graduates possess knowledge of human behavior in the social environment, the social welfare system, research and evaluation. They have well-developed basic interviewing, assessment, and helping skills. This strong academic and skill base allows BSW graduates to concentrate on information specific to the job for which they are hired. These factors plus the Child Welfare Sequence are producing a public child welfare worker with the potential to become effective faster and remain in the agency longer than workers hired from other backgrounds.

Although a social work student's primary role during the internship is that of learner, students have also completed a significant amount of work for the public child welfare agency. Their presence in the agency relieves overburdened staff of administrative and caseload responsibilities that are both within the intern's capabilities and a necessary part of the learning process. Each social work student is required to complete a semester project that is of value to the agency. Recent interns have organized a Parents Anonymous Program in a community which had none, developed an evaluation instrument for worker facilitated parent support groups, and translated official agency correspondence into Spanish. The agency's investment in the training of BSW interns has resulted in high returns in intern workload productivity.

The university has benefited from the partnership by having additional faculty to develop new curriculum and research modules on family preservation, permanency planning, and adoption. The linkages with current CPS social workers and supervisors have provided invaluable experiences for faculty and the students they teach. The clear connection with the real world of child welfare is enabling university faculty to educate prepared and skilled BSW professionals.

Using Holloway and Brager's (1985) framework, the process evaluation has provided us with case studies of personal behavioral change, structural change, and technological change. Agency supervisors and university faculty can cite numerous examples of differences in worker's attitudes toward their clients and their perspectives on the challenging work they do. There are more social work supervisors in the regions, and the decision-making process parallels the systems perspective and ethics guidelines taught in the social work curriculum. New workers who have participated in the Child Welfare Sequence start work familiar with technology and interested in innovative programs.

OUTCOME EVALUATION

The university-agency partnership has touched the lives of more than 800 students in the last ten years. For all students there was a brief exposure to a curriculum module focusing on child welfare practice. Approximately 180 students have completed internships related to child welfare, and 149 students have completed internships at CPS and have signed a formal contract to complete at least one-year of employment at CPS. In 1992, the focus was narrowed to the public child welfare agency for the internship, but students were not required to accept employment. Since 1995, students have been required to accept employment at CPS upon completion of the internship.

Tables 1-3 show the tracking results for the last ten years. Table 1 presents the demographics of the child welfare stipend recipients. Although the recipients were primarily female, they did represent the ethnic diversity of the region. The agency was particularly pleased with the number of Spanish-speaking recipients. More than 79% of the applicants were hired upon completion of the internship, and only 10% were not hired. Eight percent had their obligation to work deferred until they completed graduate school. The remaining 2% are paying back the stipend. Both the university and the agency are comfortable with these percentages because they view the internship as an important opportunity to screen job applicants for suitability of employment. More than half of those who were hired stayed beyond their commitment. The length of employment ranged from one to nine years.

In addition to the outcome tracking data collected thus far, several other evaluation initiatives that focus on longer term outcomes are underway. We have selected a random sample of current child welfare workers who received social work degrees and participated in the Title IV-E training and compared them with child welfare workers of similar experience but without social work degrees. We are examining whether there are areas where social workers preformed better than non-social workers. For the evaluation we are using the an-

TABLE 1. Demographics of Child Welfare Stipend Recipients 1989-99 (N = 149)

Demographics	*Number*	*Percent*
Male	11	7%
Female	138	93%
African American	13	9%
Hispanic	55	37%
Anglo	79	53%
Other	2	1%

TABLE 2. Hiring Data for Child Welfare Stipend Recipients (n = 149)

Hired	118	79.2%
Not Hired	16	10.7%
Nor Required/Grad. School	12	8.1%
Pay Back	3	2.0%

TABLE 3. Cumulative Longevity of Those Hired: 1989-1999

Percent Who Stayed Beyond Commitment	56%
Range of Years Employed	1 to 9 years
Highest Number of Years Employed	9 years

nual evaluation of worker performance completed by supervisors. The evaluation looks at nine areas of job performance: job knowledge; quality of work; productivity; planning; follow-up; initiative; use of supervision; use of time; and human relations. Like the exploratory study by Hopkins, Mudrick, and Rudolph (1999), this study has produced preliminary information that is consistent with what has been observed and recorded in the process evaluation, but there are still many unanswered questions, particularly about organizational and agency change.

The pilot of this evaluation tool showed that overall the differences in supervisor's ratings of workers did not vary a great deal by education. We are looking at some possible explanations for this result and examining alternative ways to look at quality of work using some new research by Glisson and Hemmelgarn (1998) that looks at the effects of organizational climate and interorganizational coordination on the quality and outcomes of children's service systems. We are also conducting a more in depth study by doing an item analysis of all of the questions that comprise each of the nine areas. There are concerns about the views of the raters being affected by whether or not they possess a social work degree. The plan for the future is to refine both the instrument and the methodology and then conduct a statewide comparison of Title IV-E prepared social workers and non-social workers. Perceptions of clients as to the quality of service they received as well as perceptions of the social workers and their supervisors will be included in the statewide comparison of the Title IV-E prepared social workers and non-social workers.

RECOMMENDATIONS FOR THE FUTURE

Tracking process and outcome evaluation results for university/agency partnerships that prepare students for public child welfare is not easy, but it is essential. We offer five key recommendations to other university-agency partnerships:

- Collaborate with all your partners at every step of the process from designing and implementing the project to evaluating it.
- Have a flexible evaluation plan that includes both process and outcome measures. Be willing to use different evaluation instruments (face-to-face interviews, e-mail surveys, telephone surveys, focus groups, written questionnaires, etc.) to obtain relevant information in the least obtrusive manner.
- Identify and control for (whenever possible) organizational factors when evaluating retention and work performance. Incorporate questions related to organizational climate and workload into your evaluation instruments.
- Identify and control for (whenever possible) individual factors when evaluating retention and work performance. Train evaluators to be unbiased and whenever possible use outside evaluators.
- Take evaluation seriously and plan well. Evaluate what you can evaluate even if you are not able to evaluate everything you want during the beginning stages. Evaluation involving partnerships is an evolutionary process.

These recommendations all require that your partnership is strong. Partnership is an easy word to say, but it is a difficult relationship to establish and maintain. The best way to begin is to start close to home, with the people you know and with whom you have worked. Start with the field supervisors who have supervised your students and have a relationship with your program. From there, build relationship with regional administrators and state-level contacts. You need to have a solid base and good relationships where you can explore the benefits of a partnership for all parties. Get input from current students, recent graduates, practitioners, and faculty.

When you have your potential partners together, you can begin the process evaluation by developing a list with three columns, one labeled with a minus sign, one with a check mark, and one with a plus sign. After you present the columns, spend a lot of time listening. Your partners will immediately volunteer suggestions for the minus column; it is easy to tell about what isn't working well. You may have to ask about what is simply working and what is working well. From this point, develop short-term and long-term goals and strategies. You can likely use some of the items in the check mark and plus sign columns to help ameliorate some of the problems identified in the minus column.

Process evaluation must be grounded in well-conceived assumptions that are developed collaboratively by all the stakeholders. It is essential that process evaluation be an ongoing process because it lays the foundation for the outcome evaluation. A process evaluation can be extremely important for child welfare partnerships because it provides up-to-date information about what services are being provided, who is being served, and the satisfaction of the students, graduates, field supervisors, agency personnel, and faculty. A process evaluation gives you important information that can be used to make ongoing improvements.

Outcome evaluations that extend beyond tracking as reported in this study are essential for the future. In the meantime, however, we need to collect and report to the public the results of the tracking outcomes that are available thus far. Many universities have this data or could access this data, and they need to share it with the public. As university-agency partnerships collectively report this data, we will have valuable information as a first step in showing the results of funding from Section 426 and Title IV-E.

This paper has reported the process and outcome evaluation results of a ten-year collaborative effort to prepare social work students for child welfare. Although the results of this partnership project are only from a case study of one Texas university and have limitations for generalizability, this beginning effort is a first step in understanding and documenting the role of social work education in preparing child welfare workers. It is hoped that these lessons learned will assist other programs to design process and outcome evaluations that study additional topics for longer periods with larger cohorts of students.

REFERENCES

Alperin, D. E. (1998). Factors relating to student satisfaction with child welfare field placements. *Journal of Social Work Education. 34 (1)*: 43-54.

Baer, B. & McLean, A. (1994). *A report: Child welfare curriculum in accredited BSW programs*. Green Bay: University of Wisconsin Social Work Program.

Dhooper, S. S., Royse, D. D., & Wolfe, L. C. (1990). Does social work education make a difference? *Social Work, 35 (1)*, 57-61.

Glisson, C. & Hemmelgarn, A. (1998). The effects of organizational climate and interorganizational coordination on the quality and outcomes of children's service systems. *Child Abuse and Neglect*, 22 (5), 401-421

Hollandsworth, S. (1998). No one knows what could be happening to those kids. *Texas Monthly 27 (4)*, 114-121, 144-149.

Holloway, S. & Brager, G. (1985). Some considerations in planning organizational change. In S. Slavin (Ed.), *An introduction to human services management* (2nd ed.) (pp. 309-318). New York: The Haworth Press.

Hopkins, K. M., Mudrick, N. R., & Rudolph, C. S. (1999). Impact of university/agency partnerships in child welfare on organizations, workers, and work activities. *Child Welfare, LXXVIII (6)*, 749-773.

Leighninger, L. & Ellett, A. J. (1998). De-professionalization in child welfare: Historical analysis and implications for social work education. Paper presented at Council on Social Work Education 44th Annual Program Meeting, Orlando, Florida, March 5-8.

Lieberman, A. A., Hornby, H., & Russell, M. (1988). Educational backgrounds and work experiences of child welfare personnel. *Social Work, 33*, 485-489.

Pecora, P. J., Briar, K. H., & Zlotnik, J. L. (1989). Addressing the program and personnel crisis in child welfare. Silver Spring, MD: National Association of Social Workers.

Rome, S. (1994). Choosing child welfare: An analysis of social work student's career choices. Washington, DC: National Association of Social Workers.

Zlotnik, J. L. (1997). *Preparing the workforce for family-centered practice: Social work education and public human services partnerships.* Alexandria, VA: Council on Social Work Education.

Reducing Conflict
Between Child Welfare Communities

Sandra Kopels, JD, MSW
Jan Carter-Black, MSW
John Poertner, DSW

SUMMARY. Conflict is inherent in child welfare practice. This article describes a collaborative project between a public child welfare agency and a school of social work (the UFOCWL) to strengthen and improve the connections between the agency and the larger community. The collaboration focused on identifying and recognizing the diverse roles and responsibilities between the various players in the child welfare system. This paper discusses the areas in which the UFOCWL addressed the conflicts between the child welfare service delivery system and the legal, domestic violence, and substance abuse communities. By facilitating understanding of the unique concerns and contributions each child welfare player brings to the table, inherent conflicts can be reduced and managed, ultimately improving the results for vulnerable children. *[Article copies available for a fee from The Haworth Document Delivery Service: 1-800-HAWORTH. E-mail address: <getinfo@haworthpressinc.com> Website: <http://www.HaworthPress.com> © 2002 by The Haworth Press, Inc. All rights reserved.]*

KEYWORDS. Collaboration, child welfare community, conflict

Sandra Kopels is Associate Professor, Jan Carter-Black is Professor, and John Poertner is Professor, all at the School of Social Work, University of Illinois at Urbana-Champaign, 1207 W. Oregon, Urbana, IL 61801.

This project was funded in part by the Illinois Department of Children and Family Services.

[Haworth co-indexing entry note]: "Reducing Conflict Between Child Welfare Communities." Kopels, Sandra, Jan Carter-Black, and John Poertner. Co-published simultaneously in *Journal of Health & Social Policy* (The Haworth Press, Inc.) Vol. 15, No. 3/4, 2002, pp. 117-129; and: *Evaluation Research in Child Welfare: Improving Outcomes Through University-Public Agency Partnerships* (ed: Katharine Briar-Lawson, and Joan Levy Zlotnik) The Haworth Press, Inc., 2002, pp. 117-129. Single or multiple copies of this article are available for a fee from The Haworth Document Delivery Service [1-800-HAWORTH, 9:00 a.m. - 5:00 p.m. (EST). E-mail address: getinfo@haworthpressinc.com].

117

> Child welfare is difficult and complicated . . . wrought with uncertainties and dilemmas. Decisions can literally mean the difference between life and death for children, and disruption or preservation of families. (Rycus and Hughes, 1994)

Conflict is inherent in child welfare practice. The conflict begins when someone has a concern about a child or family and contacts a public child welfare agency responsible for child protection. The agency investigates and if necessary, intervenes in the family situation by removing the child from the home and/or providing child welfare services to family members. The intervention may include court proceedings that can result in legally terminating the family relationship. Family members are often antagonistic towards what they believe to be unnecessary and unjustified intrusions into their lives and how they choose to raise their families. They often resent the explicit or implicit messages that there is something wrong with their parenting abilities.

In addition to conflictual relationships with families who may not want its involvement, community organizations and other social service providers often criticize public child welfare agencies. Frequently, the criticisms have revolved around issues pertaining to case decision-making by agency workers and the policies and procedures of the public child welfare organization. For example, the African-American community is critical of the fact that minority children are removed from their homes and placed in foster care at a disproportionate rate to their actual percentage of the population and are over-represented in the foster care system (O'Donnell, 1999; McRoy & Grape, 1999; Hollingsworth, 1999). Other community groups question whether government should have the right to interfere with the privacy and autonomy of the family. Because of this, decisions of child welfare professionals are often met with hostility and suspicion.

Other criticisms center around child welfare worker training and skill levels. Judges often view child welfare workers as unprepared to testify in court. Attorneys often conflict with child welfare workers regarding who should perform specific tasks when cases go to court (Stein, 1998). Questions about workers' skills, along with difficult to negotiate bureaucratic structures and a less than responsive organizational culture have been cited as problems contributing to the inadequacy of the public child welfare service delivery system (Hopkins, Mudrick, & Rudolph, 1999).

Another source of conflict relates to the roles associated with working to protect children. Historically, public child welfare workers have been perceived as "child rescuers" (Cole, 1995), focusing on saving children from abusive or neglectful families. For most child welfare workers, the protection of children is considered paramount; ensuring that children remain safe is their primary concern. For many of these families, however, child abuse is not the only factor that places them at risk. Instead, factors such as poverty, substance abuse, mental illness and domestic violence may also be present. Because of this, families are likely to encounter other social service providers who may provide services concentrating on different needs of the family. While all service providers have concerns regarding the safety of children, for certain providers, the needs of the children may not be the primary focus of service. For example, advocates for battered women mainly focus on providing shelter and support to battered women. For these advocates, the needs of the battered woman are the utmost concern; if a woman decides to stay with her abuser, domestic violence advocates support her in her choice. Typically, child protection workers do not view battered women's advocates as allies in their efforts to protect children. Rather, conflict, mistrust and non-collaboration between these groups is the rule (Findlater & Kelly, 1999).

This article describes a collaborative project between a public child welfare agency and a school of social work to strengthen and improve the connections between the child welfare agency and the larger community. The collaboration focuses on identifying and recognizing the diverse roles and responsibilities between the various players in the child welfare system. By facilitating understanding of the unique concerns and contributions each child welfare player brings to the table, inherent conflicts can be reduced and managed, ultimately improving the results for vulnerable children.

THE URBANA FIELD OFFICE CHILD WELFARE LABORATORY

The Urbana Field Office Child Welfare Laboratory (UFOCWL) resulted from a meeting between the Dean of the School of Social Work at the University of Illinois at Urbana-Champaign and the Director of the Illinois Department of Children and Family Services. They agreed to establish a collaboration, partially funded by Title IV-E, to bring child welfare practitioners and academics together on projects that would benefit the child welfare system and its clients. Additionally, the collaboration would provide a venue to educate students and faculty about public child welfare. The collaboration began with a series of meetings of staff from the two entities. Discussion centered on identifying the current challenges facing the local office of the public child welfare agency and how the resources of the school could be used to meet those challenges. What emerged from these discussions was a focus on improving the connections between the local child welfare agency and the broader communities that impact on the local child welfare agency's ability to provide children safe and permanent homes. The UFOCWL project began in January 1999 with the initial collaboration focusing on the following aspects:

- the legal system's response to child abuse and neglect (including the court system, the district attorney and police);
- the community response to families where domestic violence is present;
- the community response to families involved with substance abuse;
- the economically disadvantaged in the community who are over represented in the child welfare system;
- keeping parents connected to their children in out-of-home care;
- relationships with counseling service providers; and
- quality improvement.

The Different Communities

While the UFOCWL project targets all of the above-mentioned issues, this paper discusses the areas in which the UFOCWL addressed the conflicts between the child welfare service delivery system and the legal, domestic violence, and the substance abuse communities in Champaign County, Illinois. Consequently, initial efforts focused predominately on enhancing the relationships between organizations providing services to children and families and the legal community, with special emphasis on the issues of domestic violence and substance abuse.

For many reasons, there is great potential for conflict between a child welfare service delivery system and the legal community. First, the overall focus for social services is to support individuals, families and vulnerable groups to achieve, at the very least, a basic level of general well-being. On the other hand, the legal system is based on an adversarial system, concentrating on evidence, burdens of proof, and compliance with court mandates. Additionally, child welfare services are intervention oriented, helping families gain competencies in areas in which they may not possess the requisite skills. In contrast, the judicial system is reactive, responding only to the issues presented to the court. These divergent perspectives may contribute to the frequently observed chasm between the two domains. Some suggest the conflict lies in possible differences in "psychological preconditions" of attorneys versus social workers (Lau, 1983). Still others surmise something as rudimentary as misconceptions concerning the most appropriate role to be played during legal proceedings by each professional group (Katz, 1988). Regardless of the basis of the conflict, the child welfare system simply cannot function properly without the collaboration between the two entities (Johnson & Cahn, 1995).

Strengthening Connections with the Legal Community

This component of the collaboration project began by bringing together significant and influential members of the public child welfare agency and the legal community. The group consisted of the county's juvenile court judges, state's attorney, the executive director of the Court Appointed Special Advocates Program (CASA), senior managers of the local child welfare agency, and the project coordinators from the school of social work. The group was charged with the task of developing strategies to advance services to children and families despite the typical and seemingly inherent conflicts between the two communities. The goal for this endeavor was to enhance the relationships between the various groups involved in the child welfare system.

This goal of enhancing relationships would be accomplished by engaging in a positive, proactive, results focused, community strengths oriented dialogue with representatives of these organizations. One of the first steps was to contact the National Council of Juvenile and Family Court Judges (NCJFCJ) to assist in locating a keynote speaker for a community forum. A one day training event was held for juvenile court judges, representatives from the state's attorney's office, police officers, CASA volunteers, probation officers, privately contracted service providers and attorneys, domestic violence program advocates, substance abuse counselors and program staff, mental health workers, public and private agency child welfare workers, representatives from juvenile delinquency prevention programs, and the local ministerial alliance. The focus of the training was on maintaining children safely at home without court intervention. The training used case examples to begin discussion of developing protocols when substance abuse, domestic violence, or mental illness was the reason for involvement.

The success of this initial effort led to further dialogue between the legal community and the public child welfare agency. At subsequent planning sessions, specific procedural modifications and the clarification of roles and responsibilities were made regarding the following areas:

1. reducing the need for protective custody,
2. assessments and evaluations,
3. training needs,
4. expanded court monitors system, and
5. inter-group communication.

Reducing the Need for Protective Custody

In Illinois, a shelter care hearing is the first court appearance in cases of alleged child abuse and neglect and is held with the dual purpose of preventing families from entering into the judicial system and simultaneously ensuring that children remain safe. Under the former system, when a child was taken into protective custody, a shelter care hearing was scheduled for the morning of the following business day. The members of the collaboration determined that the scheduling of mandatory shelter care hearings should be extended to use the maximum 48-hour time period as allowed by Illinois law. By extending the time between taking protective custody and the shelter care hearing, a more thorough exploration of reasonable efforts could be made by the child protection investigator. Additionally, the change in the scheduling of the hearing could also facilitate arrangement of alternative voluntary placements that could prevent the necessity of taking protective custody. At the same time, the roles to be played by the public and private agency child welfare workers, the state's attorney's office, and the courts during the protective custody and other evidentiary hearings were clarified.

Assessments and Evaluations

All of the players involved were concerned that the particular needs of a family be properly identified and that appropriate interventions provided to the family members.

For example, in many cases, a substance abuse assessment may reveal the need for more in-depth treatment. Particular attention was given to furthering the efficiency and effectiveness of obtaining comprehensive substance abuse assessments. A strategy was developed whereby a chemical dependency assessment would be conducted immediately following the court hearing in which the assessment was ordered. The substance abuse counselor would meet the client at the local child welfare office to conduct the assessment on the day that the assessment was ordered. The resulting process reduced the frustration experienced by clients attempting to fulfill multiple tasks delineated in their service plan and ensured that the assessments were done in a timely manner that was not present prior to the strategy. Additionally, the procedures, timelines, and delineation of responsibilities for the public and private child welfare workers, state's attorney's office, consulting psychologists, substance abuse counselors and the courts were reiterated during the planning sessions.

Training Needs

Another crucial component addressed by this project were the deficits in the training programs for child welfare workers. This was especially true for the local, private child welfare agencies under contract with the public child welfare agency. These smaller, private agencies were experiencing rapid turnover of both worker and supervisory staff. Accordingly, a number of training topics were identified. These included legal screening, juvenile law and procedure, testifying in court, critical decision-making, terminating parental rights, permanency goals, client service plans, and administrative case reviews. The project members decided that the same core clinical practice training should be offered to both public and private agency child welfare workers. A joint training opportunity would contribute to an improved working relationship between these two groups as well as enhance the consistency and continuity of services to clients. In September 1999, a joint training was held, addressing many of the above-mentioned topics, with presentations made by a juvenile court judge, a state's attorney, a private attorney and an attorney for the public child welfare agency. A second training on testifying in court, with role-playing between attorneys and public and private child welfare workers was held in September 2000. This training included opportunity for child welfare workers to practice court testimony skills in direct examination and cross examination in interactive sessions with local attorneys.

Another opportunity to provide on-going training to child welfare workers took advantage of an already established education partnership between the state child welfare agency and several schools of social work within the states. The education partnership "field teachers" provide consultation to public child welfare agency workers in the areas of assessment, service planning, intervention, evaluation services, clinical skills instruction on an individual basis, and assistance in the development and delivery of training. The UFOCWL project was able to tap into resources already in place for the training of local, public child welfare workers and extend them to local, private agency child welfare workers.

Expanded Court Monitors System

A court feedback reports and monitor system was developed to provide information to the public child welfare agency about case progress during juvenile courtroom proceedings concerning child abuse and neglect. Monitors, who were employees of the public child welfare agency, completed court feedback forms to provide feedback to workers and supervisors about public child welfare agency performance. Additionally, the feedback form also serves as a tool to identify and document the judge's concerns so that those concerns may be quickly and appropriately addressed. The forms are designed to track patterns and improvement in worker performance, detect problems as they arise, and implement viable solutions to those problems quickly and efficiently. The UFOCWL project suggested an increase in the number of available courtroom monitors. Accordingly, a courtroom monitor also sits in on courtroom proceedings in which smaller, private child welfare agencies under contract with the public agency provide child welfare services. In this way, these smaller, private agencies can also be tracked for worker performance and other concerns.

Inter-Group Communication

The last strategy addressed by the planning group revolved around the issue of communication. The lines of communication between the various groups of key child welfare service community players were in enough disrepair to warrant immediate intervention. The first step taken by the project participants was to convene regularly scheduled meetings between the juvenile court judges; the public child welfare agency's legal counsel, managers, and workers; appointed court monitors; and private child welfare agency workers. These meetings would permit the monitoring of compliance by all parties, identify deficiencies in performance, facilitate the recognition of improvement and achievements, and promote meaningful dialogue.

Strengthening Connections with the Domestic Violence Community

The relationship between domestic violence programs and public child welfare agencies historically has been plagued with conflict. Controversy often revolves around which client group should be targeted for the most intensive intervention efforts–the battered woman or the children who may witness and/or experience emotional and physical abuse. Additionally, conflict between these groups is heightened when the actual perpetrator of abuse (in most cases the male), is not held responsible for the harm done to the children (Kopels & Chesnut Sheridan, in press). On a local level, another point of conflict surfaced when the child welfare agency or state's attorney's office recommended to the courts that abused women's children be taken into temporary protective custody due to their "failure to protect" them from imminent harm.

The first step in reconciling the conflict between the local domestic violence program and the local public child welfare system was recognizing that the conflict experienced locally is common throughout the country. The next step entailed consultation with others who have expertise in the area of domestic violence and its impact on child maltreatment. An expert, involved with a successful domestic violence/child welfare collaboration in Minnesota (Minnesota Center Against Violence and Abuse), was invited to meet with the public child welfare agency's unit managers, the project coordinators, and other faculty from the school of social work. Among its purposes, the meeting sought viable strategies that could be employed to enhance the working relationship between domestic violence workers and child protection services workers on case decision-making and treatment planning.

Following the meeting with the consultant, the next step was to begin dialogue with key players involved in the provision of services to battered women and their children. The police department, domestic violence advocates, representatives from the public child welfare agency, the school of social work, substance abuse program counselors, crisis nursery, and private counseling agencies were invited to participate in regularly scheduled discussion groups.

With the topic of domestic violence and child maltreatment as the primary focus of the discussions, this group worked to jointly develop a definition of domestic violence and to articulate the issues that arise in cases of domestic violence where children are involved. The group agreed there was a need to understand the multiple approaches taken by different professions and developed a domestic violence task force. While the task force began to set the agenda for their efforts, the UFOCWL project staff began compiling domestic violence protocols from around the country. The information was assembled into a handbook that was made available to service providers as a resource (Shim & Poertner, 1999).

The task force utilized a "grand rounds" concept for bringing various professions together at regular intervals to locate gaps and overlapping services in the community's response to these problems. The domestic violence and child maltreatment work group developed a set of best practice principles to respond to cases involving domestic violence and child maltreatment. These practice principles cover a number of critical procedures and services provided by various organizations and include the following:

1. The availability of a child advocate and/or counselor for children living in violent households;
2. access to short-term crisis nursery services for children aged birth through five years;
3. protocols for contacting child protection services workers in domestic violence cases when police officers use the crisis nursery for young children;
4. assessment and counseling for both the victims and perpetrators of domestic violence; and
5. interviewing, disseminating information, and aiding in development of safety plans for women who may be at risk for domestic violence.

The group's long-term goal is to create a coordinated community approach to the interrelated problems of domestic violence and child maltreatment and to develop a community-wide protocol for uniformly responding to domestic violence and child abuse.

Strengthening Connections with the Substance Abuse Community

Alcoholism and substance abuse contributes yet another layer of complexity and conflict with the child welfare system. Addiction counselors frequently advocate for keeping a family intact during a parent's addiction recovery process. They believe the disruption that accompanies the out-of-home placement of children undermines the potential for a successful outcome of abstinence for the recovering adult (Karoll & Poertner, 1999). In contrast, the child welfare system is concerned with children's safety while parents attempt to address their addictions. Child welfare advocates often recommend that children be removed from unstable or unsafe homes until the parent recovers. This conflict is heightened by the provisions of the Adoption and Safe Families Act of 1997 (P.L. 105-89), which requires states to consider permanency planning and begin termination of parental rights proceedings sooner than in the past. The effect of this law on parents with substance abuse problems is that they will have less time and more pressure to address their substance addiction before court proceedings to terminate parental rights are initiated.

Additionally, the recovery community is critical of what they perceive as the child welfare system's inadequate knowledge of the affects of substance abuse on families. They contend that addiction has an overarching effect and directly impacts on every aspect of the family system. Recognition of the actual impact of addiction on the family results in a concentrated recovery intervention aimed at assisting the entire family system (Karoll & Poertner, 1999). Further, it has been suggested that women who are substance addicted have certain unique gender-specific issues that frequently surface and are not adequately addressed (Karoll & Poertner, 1999). Given the predominance of female-headed single parent families that receive child welfare services, the system must be attuned to the special concerns of substance-addicted women.

The UFOCWL project began to address these concerns by investigating the research on drug and alcohol addicted women. The project compiled information and suggestions for training that would better prepare workers to intervene in cases involving substance addicted women and their children. They developed best practice principles for working with alcohol and substance abuse mothers which were distributed to child welfare workers for use as a basis for guiding child welfare workers towards a more informed perspective on these issues (Karoll & Poertner, 1999).

The UFOCWL project then turned towards identifying criteria used when making recommendations to the courts to reunite families across professions. A research study, currently in progress, was launched to discover the indicators professionals from various fields look for when asked to make a recommendation concerning reunification. Chemical dependence counselors, private child welfare workers, and members of the legal community, including juvenile court judges and guardian ad litems, comprised focus groups to ascertain the most salient and prevalent indicators used by a given group of service providers.

The data to be obtained from this research will produce important information that will allow the child welfare, addiction, and legal communities to understand more fully what the other groups deem as necessary conditions before they are willing to recommend and approve the reunification of a substance affected family. By clarifying these differing viewpoints about expectations for families, conflicts will be reduced. At the same time, services for families, such as permanency planning, service plans, interventions, and evaluations of progress towards desired outcomes, will be improved.

LESSONS LEARNED FROM THE PROJECT

While the UFOCWL project is ongoing and evolving, a number of pointers learned from this collaboration can be shared in order to reduce conflict between the public child welfare system and the larger community.

First, the attitudes brought to the table by the different groups must be managed. Often, the historical relationships between the numerous key players may be conflictual. The hostilities and animosities that may have characterized the working relationships of the various service providers can inhibit progress towards improving services if they are allowed to surface through a rehashing of old wounds. Adopting an attitude of working together on resolving differences and a willingness to move on in a productive and solution-focused manner is crucial. The coordinators of any such collaborative effort must create a positive, cooperative, forward looking, and solution oriented entity.

Second, the vulnerability of at-risk families is frequently heightened by the experience of being besieged by multiple and sometimes chronic problems. Therefore, any successful intervention must be multi-solution oriented, which often requires that services be coordinated across several agencies at any given time. Consequently, any collaborative effort must recognize that there are multiple key players who should be invited to the table. These players will represent varying disciplines, with diverse perspectives, and differing strategies for reaching the same goal of improving services for families and their children.

Third, the very nature of collaboration between different agencies, organizations, and professions implies equity. Care must be given to maintaining a balance between fulfilling the instrumental tasks necessary for goal attainment with the leadership tasks that aid in establishing group cohesion, loyalty, and goodwill. An assigned leader typically manages these tasks. However, participants must make critical decisions such as what will be addressed, when, how, and by whom, without the usual deference to certain individual's authority or position in the community. These kinds of collaborations may be quite tenuous unless the participants perceive they are treated fairly and respectfully.

Fourth, the attitude of the public child welfare administrator towards reducing conflict is crucial to the success of an undertaking of this magnitude. Fortunately, in the UFOCWL project, the public child welfare administrators on the state and local levels adopted the stance of reaching out to the community. They offered the agency's resources and services as a source of support and cooperation and acted as partners in the provision of services to children, families, and the community. Consequently, it seems quite possible that with time and continued effort, the conflict between the child welfare agency and the broader community may be reduced. The historical perception by the community that the public child welfare agency's role is that of the "child rescuer" may be replaced by the role of "community resource."

Finally, the single, most important lesson learned through this collaboration effort was the value of creating a set of best practice principles for and by each community involved in the provision of services to children and families. This strategy served a critical two-fold function. First, the nature of developing best practices principles as a joint effort opened up dialogue in an organized, goal-driven environment. Second, the process of developing strategies across disciplines, organizations, and agencies using a model of cooperation and collaboration, created and strengthened connections between the public child welfare agency and its surrounding service and support community.

REFERENCES

Cole, E. S. (1995). Becoming family centered: Child welfare's challenge. *Families in Society, 76,* (3), 163-172.

Findlater, J. E. and Kelly, S. (1999). Child protective services and domestic violence. The future of children: Domestic violence and children, 9 (3), 84-96. Los Altos, CA: David and Lucile Packard Foundation.

Hollingsworth, L. D. (1999). Symbolic interactionism, African American families, and the transracial adoption controversy. *Social Work, 44* (5), 443-451.

Hopkins, K. M., Mudrick, N. R. and Rudolph, C. S. (1999). Impact of university/agency partnerships in child welfare on organizations, workers, and work activities. *CHILD WELFARE, LXXVIII,* (6), 749-773.

Johnson, P. and Cahn, K. (1995). Improving child welfare practice through improvements in attorney-social worker relationships. *CHILD WELFARE, LXXIV,* (2), 383-394.

Karoll, B. R. and Poertner, J. (1999). *Women, alcoholism and child welfare workers.* Urbana, Illinois: University of Illinois at Urbana-Champaign, School of Social Work.

Katz, L. (1988). *Seeing kids through to permanence: Courtwise.* Seattle, WA: Northwest Resource Center for Children, Youth and Families.

Kopels, S. and Chesnut Sheridan, M. (in press). Adding legal insult to injury: Battered women, their children and the failure to protect. *Affilia.*

Lau, J. (1983). Lawyers vs. social workers: Is cerebral hemisphericity the culprit? *Child Welfare, LXII,* 21-27.

McRoy, R. G. and Grape, H. (1999). Skin color in transracial and inracial adoptive placements: Implications for special needs adoptions. *CHILD WELFARE, LXXVIII,* (5), 673-694.

O'Donnell, J. M. (1999). Involvement of African American fathers in kinship foster care services. *Social Work, 44,* (4), 428-441.

Rycus, J. and Hughes, R. (1994). *Child welfare competencies.* Columbus, Ohio: Institute for Human Services.

Shim, W. and Poertner, J. (1999). *Best practice: Domestic violence and child abuse and neglect.* Urbana, Illinois: University of Illinois at Urbana-Champaign, School of Social Work.

Stein, T. J. (1998). *Child welfare and the law* (Rev. ed.). Wash. DC: Child Welfare League of America Press.

An Evaluation
of Child Welfare Design Teams
in Four States

Dawn Anderson-Butcher, PhD
Hal A. Lawson, PhD
Carenlee Barkdull, MSW

SUMMARY. Empowerment-oriented design teams were structured in four states to promote collaborative practices among professionals and former clients. These teams were structured to serve as both learning and training systems, and they identified competencies for collaborative practices. Because these design teams represent a new learning and improvement system for child welfare and related service systems, and because these systems need more effective approaches to learning, training, and improvement, outcomes-oriented evaluations are imperative. The outcomes evaluation reported here relied on two evaluation strategies. First, 48 design team members completed follow-up surveys; these surveys explored individuals' perceptions of their design team involvement. Second, 22 design team members were interviewed directly; they were asked questions about the benefits and accomplishments resulting from their design team experience. These data from both evaluation strategies indicate that design teams promoted family-centered practice and interprofessional collaboration; enhanced service delivery

---

Dawn Anderson-Butcher is affiliated with The Ohio State University. Hal A. Lawson is affiliated with The University at Albany, SUNY. Carenlee Barkdull is affiliated with The University of Utah.

Address correspondence to: Dawn Anderson-Butcher, 325D Stillman Hall, 1947 College Road, College of Social Work, The Ohio State University, Columbus, OH 43210.

[Haworth co-indexing entry note]: "An Evaluation of Child Welfare Design Teams in Four States." Anderson-Butcher, Dawn, Hal A. Lawson, and Carenlee Barkdull. Co-published simultaneously in *Journal of Health & Social Policy* (The Haworth Press, Inc.) Vol. 15, No. 3/4, 2002, pp. 131-161; and: *Evaluation Research in Child Welfare: Improving Outcomes Through University-Public Agency Partnerships* (ed: Katharine Briar-Lawson, and Joan Levy Zlotnik) The Haworth Press, Inc., 2002, pp. 131-161. Single or multiple copies of this article are available for a fee from The Haworth Document Delivery Service [1-800-HAWORTH, 9:00 a.m. - 5:00 p.m. (EST). E-mail address: getinfo@haworthpressinc.com].

131

and an understanding of co-occurring needs; and fostered personal growth and self-awareness among participants. These commonalties and similarities were surprising and interesting because design teams in the four states proceeded differently. These findings are discussed in relation to emergent theory on collaborative learning processes and products. *[Article copies available for a fee from The Haworth Document Delivery Service: 1-800-HAWORTH. E-mail address: <getinfo@haworthpressinc.com> Website: <http://www.HaworthPress.com> © 2002 by The Haworth Press, Inc. All rights reserved.]*

KEYWORDS. Child welfare, empowerment-oriented education and training, collaborative practices, co-occurring needs, evaluation

When Temporary Assistance to Needy Families (TANF) replaced Aid to Families with Dependent Children (AFDC), a revolutionary policy change occurred. New strategies were needed for working with families receiving public assistance. For example, TANF's time limits and its employment and training requirements posed new challenges, both for vulnerable families and for the service providers who serve them (e.g., Briar-Lawson, 1998; 2001).

At the same time, knowledge and understanding grew about the co-occurring needs of individuals and families. The original conception of co-occurring needs became popular in psychiatry and clinical psychology. Research indicated that mental health needs and substance abuse problems tend to co-occur (e.g., Kessler, Nelson et al., 1996; Kessler, Gillis-Light et al., 1997). Once this co-occurring relationship was discovered and given the label "co-morbidity," practice challenges were identified. For example, dual diagnoses were required to detect these two needs and assess their development. Beyond the new requirements for individual practitioners, intra- and inter-system alignment challenges also have been identified (e.g., Lawson & Barkdull, 2001; U.S. Department of Human Services, 1999). Many agencies are structured to address just one need, and they frequently do not communicate with each other. For example, agencies addressing employment needs may not communicate effectively with agencies addressing substance abuse.

Recently, researchers have identified other co-occurring needs. Domestic violence as well as child abuse and neglect may accompany mental health needs and substance abuse problems (e.g., Derr & Taylor, 1999). Moreover, employment-related needs and problems, which TANF makes so important, also may be added to the list of co-occurring needs (Briar-Lawson, 2001; Briar-Lawson, Lawson et al., 1999).

Thus, revolutionary policy change such as TANF and new knowledge development about co-occurring needs implicate all levels of child welfare practice. They require changes in supervision, management, and front-line practice. In addition, they require changes in inter-agency relationships.

Upon closer inspection, the changes related to child welfare practice and policies may seem daunting. For example, with AFDC providers determined eligibility and then routinely distributed benefits; with TANF, many of these same workers must promote individual and family self-sufficiency through employment and employment-related supports. Will they be able to make this transition? What training and capacity-building supports will they need? Will TANF result in a growing tide of children and youth entering the child welfare system; and if so, what can be done to stem this tide?

Moreover, how will social and health service providers learn to assess and address the co-occurring needs of the most vulnerable families? Can professionals learn to collaborate with each other? Can they learn to collaborate with families? How? What are the barriers, constraints and facilitators for collaboration? How do local contexts influence the development of different kinds of collaboration? What designs are needed for interprofessional education and training (IPET) programs? How can preservice and professional development IPET programs respond to the diversity of local communities and avoid the limitations associated with conventional training programs? How might family-centered, child welfare collaboratives become connected to other collaboratives (e.g., school-linked collaboratives, health collaboratives, youth development collaboratives)? Daunting questions like these pose significant challenges for practice, training, learning, and systems alignment and change.

A comprehensive, complex four-state initiative was developed in response to the above questions and others. This initiative was designed to provide learning, training, and capacity-building assistance to child welfare and companion systems, which serve vulnerable children, youth, and families. It targeted multiple forms of collaboration, especially interprofessional collaboration, family-centered collaboration, and community collaboration (e.g., Lawson & Barkdull, 2001). It involved the participation of professionals, former clients (called family experts), and university professors in four states. These states were Utah, Colorado, Nevada, and New Mexico, and they were grouped together because of the similarities they enjoy by virtue of their location in the inter-mountain west. Two grants were awarded from the Children's Bureau, U.S. Department of Health and Human Services, in support of this work.[1]

The evaluation research reported here derives from this initiative. The initiative is described first. The evaluation design and data follow.

AN OVERVIEW OF THE INITIATIVE

A regional steering committee was structured to oversee the planning and evaluation design. This committee included a representative sample of university-community team members, agency heads, the university faculty training facilitators, and the principal investigators, Katharine Briar-Lawson and Hal A. Lawson. This steering committee functioned as both a governance structure and a collaborative action research team. The proposed work was, to greater or lesser degrees, new to everyone. Everyone evidenced needs for learning, social support, and technical assistance. The committee quickly became a community of practice (Wenger, 1999), i.e., a special kind of learning and development group. It served as a mechanism for learning, development, identity formation, and continuous quality improvement.

Early in its work, this steering committee developed a guiding vision, mission, objectives, values, and guiding principles. The mission was: To enable the development of family-centered, culturally-responsive, interprofessional knowledge, skills, attitudes, and values that tie the child welfare goals of child protection, permanency, and family preservation to the needs of economic self-sufficiency, mental health, domestic violence, and substance abuse; and to do so in ways that promote collaboration, service integration, and university reforms.[2]

A key challenge was to accommodate differences and uniqueness across the initial four sites, while at the same time identifying and understanding cross-state commonalties. Representatives from each state and site sought assurances that this initiative was not one that was characterized as "one size fits all in a one best system." On the other hand, it remained important to treat the initiative as a whole, one that was more than the sum of the four states that served as its component parts. An empowerment-oriented model and the idea of design teams for learning and development provided one source of uniformity.

INTRODUCING THE EMPOWERMENT-ORIENTED MODEL AND THE DESIGN TEAMS

An empowerment-oriented education and training model was a cornerstone in the original grant proposals. This new model was *suggested* by several kinds of research literature as well as by the principal investigator's direct experiences with conventional training. The word "suggested" is employed for good reason. Although the model could be described in principle, and a preliminary literature review supported its development, its complete elaboration awaited the acid tests of practice.[3]

A more complete design and implementation in practice also brought demands for an innovative, empowerment-oriented evaluation strategy. This evaluation had to accommodate this initiative's complexity and, at the same time, facilitate the continuous development of the model. Furthermore, the evaluation needed to monitor the model's effects and outcomes. If there were encouraging signs of progress, possible causal pathways and important correlations needed to be identified. At the same time, site-based differences needed to be accommodated. Contextual diversity, distance, and time-related challenges were present from the beginning.

The shift from AFDC to TANF and the challenges posed by knowledge about co-occurring needs challenged everyone to design new service delivery strategies and systems. When design challenges are omni-present, training is difficult, if not impossible. Training, strictly defined, is certainty–and stability-oriented. All of its assumptions and requirements depend on clarity and precision concerning practice requirements and systems configurations (Lawson, under review; Lawson et al., in press; Lawson, Petersen, & Briar-Lawson, 2001). In the case of this initiative, innovative practices had to be developed, and new systems configurations needed to be invented. In this initiative, new *learning designs* were prerequisite to the training that would eventuate (Lawson, 2000; Lawson, Petersen, & Briar-Lawson, 2001). Toward this end, design teams were formed in each of the four original sites (Reno, Nevada; Salt Lake City, Utah; Las Cruces, New Mexico; and Colorado Springs, Colorado).

Design teams, it shall become apparent, are action learning systems. Faculty facilitators from social work education programs were charged with forming these teams. In turn, teams were charged with designing new service delivery models, identifying competencies, and designing training and learning systems in support of new practices and systems designs.

DESIGN TEAM'S COMPOSITION AND PROCESS

A key aspect of empowerment is joint ownership, enfranchisement, and power-sharing (Lawson, 2001). The empowerment-oriented process begins when participants accept invitations issued by faculty facilitators to join permanent teams. Two groups of experts comprise the teams: (1) Family experts, i.e., persons who are experts because of their careers as "clients" in the various service systems and their experiences with co-occurring challenges involving substance abuse, mental health needs, domestic violence, and employment-related assistance and social supports; and (2) Helping professionals from relevant service sectors who are concerned with one or more of these co-occurring needs. These service sectors include domestic violence, mental health, employment and workforce services, substance abuse, juvenile and criminal justice, child and family services, and child protection services.

This label, design team, is apt for six reasons:

- the composition of the group (diverse professionals and former "clients" called family experts) represents a new design for teaching, learning, and staff development-support;
- the design team is expected to "go outside the lines" as needed to invent and pioneer service strategies that improve outcomes;
- through the empowerment-oriented training and capacity-building process, team members integrate design team strategies within their agencies and everyday practice;
- after their work is completed, team members will help other teams, in other places, design their service strategies;
- teams have designed and delivered "training" for other individuals and teams; and
- these teams may become permanent, self-managed work teams, which provide mutual support and problem-solving assistance for improved outcomes, worker retention, and organizational learning. In other words, the design teams may become part of new organizational designs for the human services.

Participatory and collaborative action research are used throughout the design team's learning and development process (Lawson, Petersen, & Briar-Lawson, 2001). In other words, teams generate data in response to questions and challenges posed by the facilitator; act on the data they generate; and, create more data as they identify competencies and create action plans. Forms of action research also generate data for a continuous, formative evaluation. In other words, evaluation is embedded in the design team process, and evaluation takes on many of the features of empowerment evaluation (Fetterman, Kaftarian, & Wandersman, 1996).

In addition to forms of action research, this design team model combines aspects of social learning (e.g., Gee & Green, 1998; Salomon & Perkins, 1998) and sociocultural learning. While social learning theory focuses on individuals, albeit in the context of the group, sociocultural theory focuses on teams, activity settings, and institutional systems.

Sociocultural learning theory mirrors the realities and demands of collaborative practice (e.g., Cole, 1997; Lawson, under review; Rogoff, 1998; Rogoff, Matusov, & White, 1996; Vygotsky, 1978). In sociocultural theory, individuals are viewed as inseparable from cultural traditions and practices, group dynamics, organizational characteristics, and the creation of new social and institutional settings. In this perspective, the design team comprises a special community of practice (Wenger, 1999). It enables individual and group learning; and as learning proceeds, the team develops strong social relationships and gains the social cohesion that characterizes healthy learning and practice communities.

Design teams, with their emphasis on collaborative action research and learning, are intended to result in permanent community teams that practice and learn together. In this sense, the design team model is intended to have high ecological validity, i.e., high correspondence between the conditions for learning and the conditions for actual practice. For example, like collaborative teams in community and school settings, design teams are structured to generate new knowledge and understanding at the same time they design practice and policy innovations (Lawson & Sailor, 2000). For example, the design teams generated competencies that others could use in training (Lawson, Petersen, & Briar-Lawson, 2001).

The focus on the team is not, however, at the expense of a focus on individuals. Individual as well as team problem-solving abilities are emphasized. Stronger, trusting interpersonal relationships are targeted in the design team process. Participants are expected to negotiate the specific details of the service strategies that will work in their local communities. By placing participants at center stage and responding to their needs, achievements, and situational constraints, opportunities for active learning, mutual teaching, and training-knowledge transfer and knowledge utilization are maximized (Lawson, Briar-Lawson, & Petersen, 2001).

To reiterate, a faculty facilitator structures participant's interactions and learning. Facilitators are "guides on the side" instead of "sages on the stage." And they are expected to learn along with participants as they facilitate and observe. In other words, conventional distinctions between trainers (as *the* experts) and trainees (who need and are present to receive, often passively, trainer's expertise) are irrelevant in this model. This claim does not deny the need for expert facilitators of training.

Facilitators in this model have other kinds of expertise (Lawson et al., in press). In this model, the facilitators play pivotal roles in helping to structure the learning and development process. They structure learning environments and provide learning experiences. The idea is for participants and the facilitator to become a community of practice (Wenger, 1999). The facilitator provides conceptual and intervention "tools" that help participants draw upon their experiences and expertise; surface and express them; receive reactions and critical feedback from others; use their collaboration to merge them into new intervention and improvement strategies upon which all can agree; and then take them into real world practice for implementation, modification and testing. This learning and development process is invaluable when experienced people are involved, and these people are expected to change. Experienced professionals are sometimes resistant to change, and they may prefer their customary routines. In addition, these routines are so well learned and internalized that they often become "tacit," that is, they are taken for granted and automatic. The design team process helps "surface" team member's routines and theories, making them explicit, public, and testable. Mutual learning and teaching occur as team members engage in purposeful dialogue that effectively tests member's pet routines and theories. This process is sometimes difficult and delicate.

Faculty facilitators and other design team members work together to structure a safe and secure learning environment for this difficult and delicate work. As the idea of "community of practice" suggests, learning and development are accompanied and facilitated by means of social supports. People feel empowered at the same time they empower others. Empowerment-oriented interactions and social supports often provide team members with the equivalent of cognitive scaffolds, which facilitate powerful learning and development.

Design teams involve collaborative action research and learning because they are structured to facilitate collaborative practices. Figure 1 provides an overview of the model's key features. This figure depicts two kinds of dialectical relationships, i.e., never-ending, healthy tensions. One tension involves design teams as learning systems and conventional training. The other involves interprofessional collaboration and family-centered collaboration. When these dialectical relationships are involved, it is not one or the other; it is one *and* the other. For example, design team's work informs and guides training. Interprofessional collaboration often informs family-centered collaboration, and vice versa.

To recapitulate, teams operated in four states. The four original design teams were structured to facilitate university-community partnerships in each state. Teams targeted systems and cross-systems learning and change. In addition, a four-state learning and development was formed, and the steering committee provided its hub. All in all, then, this was a complex change initiative. It was predicated on new assumptions, promoted innovative learning and training designs, and targeted novel service delivery configurations.

SITE-SPECIFIC DESIGN TEAM FEATURES AND STRUCTURES

These commonalties and similarities notwithstanding, the original four teams, like their respective universities and communities, exhibited several differences. For example, neighborhood-based, collaborative child welfare

FIGURE 1. An Overview of the Design Team and Its Integral Components

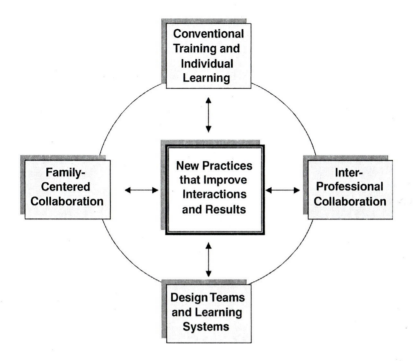

teams already were operating in Utah, so the Utah design team focused more on the importance of family experts, family-centered practice, and improved access and coordination of services. In New Mexico, the design team planned training sessions, which combined action learning and conventional training techniques. In Nevada, Nancy Petersen facilitated a design team process that resulted in an innovative learning system, an exemplary curriculum for community collaboration, and learning-training approach. The Colorado team, operating initially in Colorado Springs, selectively incorporated the Nevada materials at the same time they developed their own. At the same time, the El Paso County Department of Human Services, the site for the Colorado Springs Team, was involved with system-wide innovations involving the use of TANF to serve as the prevention arm of child welfare in support of a mission to prevent and eliminate poverty (Berns & Drake, 1999). Thus, while all four sites used the language of "design teams," upon closer inspection they were quite diverse.

This diversity increased as the scale-up process commenced. For example, scale-up design teams in Colorado were structured in First Nation Communities, rural communities, and urban communities. Although teams knew about the need to respond to policy change (e.g., the shift from AFDC to TANF), each started with different priorities and proceeded on different pathways. In Nevada, the Las Vegas site was able to start with the documented processes and achievements of the original Reno site, allowing the scale up design team to augment both the learning process and the curricular products.

To summarize: All of the sites utilized the learning systems approach represented by the design team process (Lawson, 2000; under review; Lawson, Petersen, & Briar-Lawson, 2001). All were charged with developing competencies and planning training for others. All promoted interprofessional collaboration and family-centered collaboration in support of new service delivery systems and in response to policy change and practice needs. All were mechanisms for university-community-state agency partnerships. Even so, teams had considerable discretion and autonomy, and their surrounding contexts differed significantly. Each team could be viewed legitimately as a somewhat unique case.

EVALUATION AND RELATED CHALLENGES

Complex change initiatives like this one pose formidable evaluation-related challenges. The fact that teams operated in different time frames, in different places and contexts, and with varying receptivity to evaluation added to the challenge. The original evaluation plan was developed in response to these challenges.

Design team facilitators were charged with being co-evaluators. This role is consistent with action learning and research approaches. Action research performed by team facilitators is reported elsewhere (Lawson, Petersen, & Briar-Lawson, 2001; Lawson et al., in press). Furthermore, this co-evaluator role can be extended to every design team member. In design teams, everyone is potentially a teacher and a learner; likewise, everyone is an action researcher and co-evaluator. Although this potential remained untapped, it remains an important way to address the challenges associated with complexity and diversity.

A process evaluation was launched in 1999 under the direction of one of the principal investigators (Lawson). It involved focus group interviews of design team professionals and family experts and written responses of 89 participants to a five-item questionnaire (Lawson, Briar-Lawson et al., 1999). It included a journey analysis evaluation of how the design team process may have influenced, and was influenced by, significant agency restructuring in the El Paso County Department of Human Services in Colorado Springs, Colorado (Lawson, 1999; Lawson, Khaja, & Soto, 1999). This phase also included collaborative action research in Utah with middle managers of neighborhood-based child welfare teams who also served on design teams (e.g., VanWagoner, Boyer et al., 2001).

This initial evaluation phase provided important process and product data. These data were fed back to facilitators and used to improve the design team process. For example, the micro-dynamics of design teams were depicted in a logic model (Lawson, Petersen, & Briar-Lawson, 2001). Moreover, relevant data were used in El Paso County to renew efforts aimed at organizational restructuring. Above all, this process evaluation yielded data about the micro-processes of design team dynamics, including the impact of design teams on family-centered collaboration and interprofessional collaboration (Lawson, Petersen, & Briar-Lawson, 2001). In other words, phase one data indicated that the design team process was having its intended impacts, albeit not uniformly among all design team members or in all of the sites (Lawson, Briar-Lawson et al., 1999).

The second phase of the evaluation began one and one-half years later. Mindful of needs for objectivity, the lead evaluator in this second phase (Anderson-Butcher) was contracted to assume responsibility for data collection, interpretation, and presentation. In this second phase, interest resided in the effectiveness of the design team process and model. The University of Utah's Institutional Review Board approved study procedures.

Two methods were used. First, the lead evaluator sent follow-up surveys to members of four design teams. These surveys explored member's perceptions about their involvement in their respective design teams. Participants were asked specific questions about the quality of their design team experience and its related impacts on practice. Second, the lead evaluator conducted qualitative interviews with design team members in order to elicit member's beliefs and perceptions about the benefits and accomplishments resulting from the design teams. The interviews also aimed to gain an understanding of the design team member's perceptions related to their personal experiences on design teams. These two methods yielded important data. These data are presented in two parts; each part corresponds to the method employed.

PART ONE: THE FOLLOW-UP SURVEYS

Participants

Forty-eight members of the original design teams completed questionnaires assessing the overall effectiveness of the design team process. The mean age of respondents was 47.74 years ($SD = 7.9$) and ranged from 33 to 64 years of age.

Eight were male and 40 were female. Of all respondents, 29% were family experts; 23% middle managers; 21% front-line practitioners; 11% top-level administrators; 4% university liaisons and facilitators; 4% counselors; 2% school practitioners; and 6% other. This is representative of the typical make-up of design teams, except that family expert data may be over-represented.

When respondents were asked how much they were involved in the design team, the mean response was 6.74 (*SD* = 1.83) on a scale of 1 (*not at all involved*) to 9 (*very involved*). Also, 17% of the respondents had been involved in the design team more than 2 years; 15% indicated they had been involved one to two years; 55% were involved for six months to one year; and 13% had been involved less than six months. Excluding family experts, participants had been working in human services for an average of 13 years.

Data Collection and Instrumentation

Members of the four original (and long-standing) design teams were sent a brief survey assessing the overall effectiveness of the design team process. Each of these teams had been in operation for at least nine months. A total of 79 design team members were mailed the survey and a stamped-return envelope. Forty-eight respondents completed and returned the survey, indicating a 61% response rate.

The nine items on the survey are displayed in Table 1. Responses were rated on a 5-point Likert-type scale ranging from 1 (*strongly disagree*) to 5 (*strongly agree*). The psychometric properties of this instrument are unknown.

Data Analyses and Results

Table 1 presents mean responses, medians, and standard deviations for each questionnaire item. In general, study participants had favorable opinions related to their experiences on the design team. The most favorable response among participants dealt with encouraging others to "value the input of parents and families." This positive response suggests the importance of family experts (i.e., former clients or past recipients of services) and family-centered collaboration in the design team process. Responses also were affirming for items related to collaboration and information sharing. Moreover, participants suggested that the design team had been a "valuable experience"; and that they had "learned a lot" from their participation. Less favorable responses were noted on items related to actual changes in practice.

PART TWO: QUALITATIVE INTERVIEWS

Participants

Interviews were conducted with twenty-two design team members. The sample consisted of five people from Utah, seven from Colorado, seven from

TABLE 1. Means, Medians, and Standard Deviations Describing the Value of Design Teams (n = 48)

Item	M	Mdn	SD
1. Participation in the design team has been a valuable experience for me.	3.51	4.00	.98
2. People needing help in our community have experienced greater success in achieving their goals as a result of the design team process.	2.57	3.00	.90
3. Since participating in the design team, I have collaborated more with other professionals.	3.28	4.00	1.13
4. My practice with families has positively changed since my participation in the design team.	2.82	3.00	1.10
5. I have shared information learned in the design team with other persons with whom I work.	3.54	4.00	1.05
6. I have learned a lot because of my involvement in the design team.	3.40	4.00	1.06
7. My practice with other agencies has been positively affected by my participation in the design team.	3.07	3.00	1.16
8. Since participating in the design team, I have encouraged other persons with whom I work to value the input and expertise of parents and families.	3.02	3.00	1.05
9. Since, I have encouraged others to value the input of parents and families.	3.60	4.00	1.00

Nevada, and three from New Mexico. Nine of the design team members interviewed were university-based facilitators, six were family experts, three were child welfare middle managers, two were state child welfare administrators, and two were non-child welfare front-line professionals. Sixteen were female and six were male.

Data Collection and Interview Schedule

Two years into the design team process, facilitators from Utah, Colorado, Nevada, and New Mexico identified people on their design teams to serve as key informants. Interviews were conducted with 88% of these identified design team members. Nine of the interviews were conducted face-to-face. Eleven of the interviews could not be conducted in person; they were conducted over the telephone. Each interview lasted approximately forty-five minutes.

Interviews were designed to elicit each design team member's beliefs, ideas, and opinions about their participation in their own words. An interview schedule comprised of seven open-ended, non-directive questions guided the discussion. Questions included:

a. What do you believe have been the major accomplishments of the design team(s)?
b. Has participation in the design team process changed practice or policy?
c. Have you encountered barriers and if so, what are they?
d. How did you or others involved deal with any barriers?
e. What have you learned as a result of your involvement?
f. What have been some of the high points and low points related to your involvement?
g. Can you share any lessons learned from the experience?

As is customary with qualitative interviewing, the evaluator probed for more details as participant's responded. The evaluator recorded the comments made by study participants in an interview schedule. The evaluator then transcribed these recordings immediately following the interviews.

Data Analyses and Results

The researcher reviewed the interview transcriptions for overall themes. Once familiar with the interview responses, the researcher deciphered individual quotes from each interview that represented single items or themes (Miles & Huberman, 1994). These quotes served as the raw data.

The researcher then coded the raw data into classification schemes using clustering techniques to compare and contrast the quotes. Inductive techniques were used, therefore, allowing themes to emerge from the data that were mutually exclusive and inclusive (Patton, 1990). Themes and categories were reshaped, modified, omitted, and added to other themes and categories as warranted by the raw data. This process continued until no further categories could be created.

Consensus validation was established with a peer reviewer who was familiar with the data (Lincoln & Guba, 1985). The peer reviewer correctly coded 87% of the raw data quotes; this indicates moderate to high validity. When discrepancies were found, the evaluator and the reviewer re-clustered the themes to establishing consistency.

Themes related to design team implementation and resultant outcomes emerged from the data. Only data related to design team outcomes are presented here.[4] Three higher-order themes emerged: (a) design team outcomes associated with family-centered practice;[5] (b) service delivery; and, (c) personal benefits. Figure 2 presents a flow chart examining each theme and the percentage of design team members interviewed that indicated each lower-order theme. Each theme is discussed in greater detail next.

Family-Centered Practice. Participants in the study indicated that the design team process promoted values, beliefs, and positive attitudes about family-centered practice. For instance, interviewees discussed how the design team was grounded in teaching respect for others, having equality in relationships, listening and valuing what others say, and coming from a strength-based perspective. Most of these outcomes were directly linked to the role of family experts within the design team. Three quotes from study participants highlight this importance:

> One of the major accomplishments was the family experts. They were able to provide information to professionals. They enlightened professionals and told us the things the people we work with were going through. It was what they were experiencing. They had 2-3 appointments in the same day, no one particular person knew that because the clients/family experts were reporting to so many different people. They were pulled from puller to post. . . . I became more sensitive, just being in the room with them. They were telling us what we did, could do, and should do. I was educated here.

> I have more sensitivity. It was a re-awakening. It was getting back to the way I first started in social work. If I were to go back to direct practice, I would have a different approach. "You direct me" would have been my approach with clients. Now I would ask the clients what they want out of it and together we would create the plan.

> Family experts were helpful to me. They helped me realize that I have compartmentalized some of my responsiveness (to clients). I now see this. Myself and people (participating on the design teams) have a greater sense of awareness.

Practice and policy changes related to family-centered practice also were evident. Administrators discussed new trainings and curriculums that promoted the value of family-centered practice. University faculty brought family experts to classrooms to teach students about being family-centered. Practice with families changed. In the words of two design team members:

> The intake process is better. There is better integration of child welfare and TANF. We have them in the same building. This is closer to single entity point than any other state.

> The physical nature of the building was not client-friendly. No one greets you at the door. People wondered where they go. . . . People didn't know whether to take a number, go to the counter, or wait in line. People who had appointments would take a number and then miss their appointment because they didn't know. We have changed this. Now there are signs

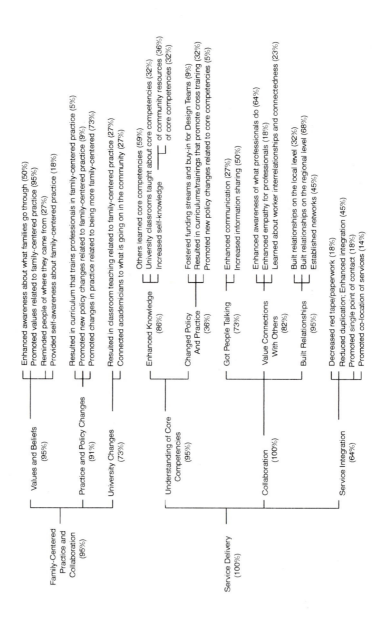

FIGURE 2. Content Analyses of Design Team Outcome-Related Themes (Parentheses Indicate Percentage of the 22 Interviewed that Noted the Theme)

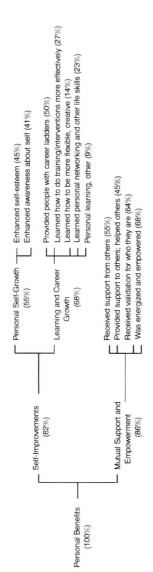

Personal Benefits (100%)

Self-Improvements (82%)

Personal Self-Growth (55%)
— Enhanced self-esteem (45%)
— Enhanced awareness about self (41%)

Learning and Career Growth (68%)
— Provided people with career ladders (50%)
— Learned how to do training/interventions more effectively (27%)
— Learned how to be more flexible, creative (14%)
— Learned personal networking and other life skills (23%)
— Personal learning, other (9%)

Mutual Support and Empowerment (86%)
— Received support from others (55%)
— Provided support to others; helped others (45%)
— Received validation for who they are (64%)
— Was energized and empowered (68%)

147

over each place that tell people where to go. They are thinking about putting a desk around the front door just for information. Then people can ask questions.

Service Delivery. Study participants noted many design team outcomes related to enhanced service delivery. First, study participants identified that their own knowledge and practice related to core competencies were enhanced. For instance, individuals working in child welfare noted that they learned about core competencies and practice related to TANF, domestic violence, substance abuse, and mental health. On the other hand, professionals working in non-child welfare-related fields became more aware of laws and policies related to child welfare. Similarly, study participants noted that university classrooms were teaching students about these core practice areas, emphasizing the co-occurrence of needs and problems within family systems. It was proposed by some study participants that these "up and coming" social workers would graduate from their academic programs better prepared to work with families in need.

Some study participants noted that the design team they participated on identified core competencies for all workers and incorporated them into their systems. In other words, these core competencies, developed by and through design teams, became defining features of optimal practice.

For instance, TANF workers and Department of Family Service's workers now are cross-trained in some agencies. Funding streams for child welfare and eligibility have been merged to maximize service delivery for families. Moreover, resource manuals describing the signs and symptoms of each competency area were provided to employees to guide their practice with families. Practice changes also were noted. According to one design team member:

> I have found that eligibility workers are more cued in on domestic violence and substance abuse relationships . . . that there is a co-occurring need. They are using words and language that they haven't done in eight years. They are asking the right questions to look at interrelationships.
>
> Forms filed out by child welfare professionals have been changed to ensure communication. Instead of saying "Is there another worker?" The form now asks "Have you had a conversation with the other worker about this case?" Things are more concrete. It now asks "Have you discussed plans with" or "Have you talked with (the other worker)."

Furthermore, collaboration and communication networks were strengthened through the design team process. The design teams built relationships among service providers, which in turn enhanced service delivery. Study participants noted that people and agencies were now talking that never had. New relationships, networks, and supports were created.

Moreover, a sense of connection and interdependence among design team members developed. Team members gained an understanding of the importance of each other's jobs in serving vulnerable children and families. One participant summarizes:

> I saw the coming together of people. Many didn't know what services were available. What happened in the design team was that there was information dissemination between people. They realized that there was duplication of service areas . . . that people and agencies were doing the same things. They basically learned who else was in town. . . . It was a get acquainted type of thing. People learned what was there in the community. There was sharing and communication.

This communication enhanced practice and service integration. For example, one family expert noted:

> The Department of Human Services (DHS) and TANF were in two different buildings. Now we have three people from DHS who have moved to the TANF offices. It's more family-friendly now. For example, if someone in the office needs this, they used to call three different people. Not anymore. . . . There are now three workers over there who can help.

Furthermore, relationships on multiple levels were built through the design team process. Specifically:

- child welfare workers developed relationships with non-child welfare-related professionals;
- family experts developed relationships with service providers;
- university faculty members developed relationships with family experts, social service providers, and both community and state administrators; and
- top level administrators developed relationships with front-line practitioners, family experts, and social work education faculty.

Furthermore, relationships were developed at the regional level. For instance:

- design team facilitators from the four states developed friendships and support systems;
- middle managers and front-line practitioners from some states shared ideas and practice strategies with design team members in other states;
- administrators from some states brainstormed with other administrators in the region about policy and creative funding strategies; and

- university faculty developed working relationships with administrators and policy-makers within the region.

In brief, many networks developed. These support networks and the working teams that derived from them were the direct result of the design team process.

Personal Benefits. The final higher order theme noted by the study participants dealt with outcomes related to self-growth, career advancements, personal learning, and the experience of mutual support and empowerment. The study participants told us that the design team process was empowering and validating. One family expert stated:

> I got my self-esteem back. A lot of it. It changed my attitude about my self. I went from an addict to a person of worth. The design team helped me make this change, they always listened, there was no judgment, no one pointed fingers at me. . . . They were the only people I have ever met that were like that.

Professionals concurred. One child welfare middle manager noted:

> The design team opened a whole new world for me. I practiced in my own world, my world of direct practice, or of exploring community. I never saw myself as a leader, that I had something others could learn from. People in the design team acknowledged my strengths. This was very affirming. Part of me never was confident in this. I know I can now. I am someone who knows something.

Many professionals and non-professionals experienced career enhancements because of their design team experience. Agency people learned new strategies that would make them more effective in their current positions. Design team members were promoted within their agencies, or recruited out of their agencies by other design team members. Family experts have gone back to school, found jobs in human services, and written books about their past life experiences. One family expert even noted that her resume "looked really good" because it included her design team involvement.

DISCUSSION

It is important to ground the findings from these two evaluation methods within the context of the design team mission and purpose. To reiterate, the mission is: To enable the development of family-centered, culturally-responsive, interprofessional knowledge, skills, attitudes, and values that tie child welfare goals to other co-occurring needs present within families; and to do so in ways that promote collaboration, service integration, and university reforms. In response, university-community partnerships were developed that created new service delivery strategies and training/learning systems. The study findings indicate that the design teams accomplished these missions and purposes.

First, both evaluation strategies found that the design teams had significant impacts on promoting family-centered practice (Lawson & Barkdull, 2001). For instance, 95% of the design team members interviewed noted that the design team enhanced attitudes, values, and beliefs about family-centered practice. Likewise, design team members surveyed strongly indicated that since their participation, they had "encouraged others to value the input of parents and families." Family experts played a pivotal role on the design teams. For example, when they informed professionals about what hurt and what helped, professionals had to examine their practice theories and their agencies' practices. This fresh perspective was an important part of this design team process.

Similarly, professionals learned that family experts had important knowledge that they (the professionals) did not have, but needed. Family experts helped professionals expand their knowledge bases, and they helped professionals gain future commitments to gain more such knowledge from the individuals and families they serve. Few professionals left the design team process with the assumption that many brought–namely, that professional knows best and the people in need are merely dependent clients. This new orientation represents a different style of professionalism called social trustee, civic professionalism (Lawson, 2001), and it involves citizen professionals serving and empowering other citizens.

Team members described their new and renewed commitments to parents and families as family-centered practice. In contrast, the design team model is structured to develop commitments to family-centered collaboration (e.g., Lawson & Barkdull, 2001). Because clear distinctions exist between family-centered practice and family-centered collaboration, team member's references to family-centered practice is an interesting finding. At least four interpretations of this finding are plausible, and they are not mutually exclusive.

First, this distinction is rather new; it is not institutionalized in textbooks, curricular materials, and daily practices. In other words, while the concept (and language) of family-centered practice is institutionalized, the concept (and language) of family-centered collaboration is not. Second, faculty facilitators may not have emphasized this distinction with team members. Third, this distinction may not be important to team members, or to facilitators. That is, they may be using a different concept (family-centered practice), but they have in mind the meanings and practices associated with family-centered collaboration. And fourth, these design teams may not have been powerful enough, under the terms and conditions surrounding their operation, to persuade team members to proceed beyond family-centered practice to the profound power-sharing and related changes associated with family-centered collaboration.

Unfortunately, this evaluation did not include probes into this interesting and important area of learning, training, and practice. Nor did it include observations of team member's work practices, which is arguably the most important way to determine the relationship between team member's espoused commitments and practice theories and their actual theories in use (e.g., Argyris & Schön, 1996). Future evaluations and research should attend to this interesting and important anomaly.

Design teams were structured to promote practice and policy changes, and members indicated that teams were successful, at least to some extent. For example, respondents identified three related kinds of service delivery changes:

   a. changes in front line practice and in administration;
   b. changes in community and university systems; and
   c. changes in the relationship among diverse professionals and recipients of services.

These changes are suggestive of complex change involving systems and inter-system relations.

Second, findings suggest that service delivery was enhanced. Survey respondents strongly indicated that they "learned a lot" because of their involvement in the design teams. Interview data provide evidence of what design team members learned. They learned core competencies at the same time they developed them. And they learned about community resources and how to access them. Design team members also learned about the key indicators of co-occurring needs, especially needs for which they had received little or no previous training. For example, referral was facilitated. Design team members learned "who to call" and "where to go" to support the families with multiple needs. Students at the university also learned these competencies in their classrooms. In other words, the design team promoted changes in social work education curricula that were more responsive to teaching the skills, knowledge areas, and values that were needed within the practice field.

Furthermore, both survey and interview responses suggest that the design team process enhanced collaboration among service providers. New relationships were built, communication was enhanced, information was shared, and people began to value the new connections they developed through the design team process. Thanks to family experts, professionals learned how important it is not to overwhelm clients by duplicating services and supports. Thus, design teams played an important role in expanding on case plans, and further supporting families with multiple needs and fostering their growth and development.

The final theme was an indirect outcome associated with participation in the design teams. It is related to the compelling effect of the design team process on building capacity, supporting, empowering, and validating practitioners, while enhancing self-esteem and awareness. The design team process prioritizes mutual support, emphasizes equal "playing fields," and values all participants as human beings first; and then secondarily for their work roles, agency sponsorships, and, in the case of family experts, their prior histories. Unlike training, which emphasizes technical-procedural competence, design teams focus on people's meaning systems and identities, assuming an intricate and important relationship between who people are and what they do.

In this perspective, it is important that team members, professionals, faculty facilitators, and family experts alike, cited personal benefits and even profound transformations that occurred through the design team process (see also Lawson et al., in press). Changes like these are related to the meaning and quality of one's work and work environment. These changes may be one key to improved practices for worker recruitment and retention. The design team process is intended to result in permanent work teams that routinely engage in collaboration, in turn improving the well-being of workers and the quality of their workplaces (Lawson & Barkdull, 2001). Although this evaluation did not explore all such benefits, its findings signal promising possibilities.

Family experts involved on the design teams described many of the same identity- and meaning-related benefits cited by professionals. The family experts also felt validated and supported. For instance, one parent stated, "Me and the others learned that no matter where you are at, we all slip up and screw up. The design team made it quite clear that you were still welcome. There was unconditional concern and care." Another stated, "It really helped my self-esteem to be a part of a group like that. . . . I felt very important in that the state and the county were reaching out and trying to understand." Moreover, three family experts interviewed were able to use their design team experience to find employment. This finding is a serendipitous effect of the design team process, and it merits future exploration.

In summary, design teams are associated with multiple benefits and desirable outcomes. Higher order themes related to benefits include enhanced family-centered practice and collaboration, service delivery, and personal growth. The design team members that participated in the two evaluations told evaluators that these benefits were accrued (a) across design teams (i.e., in all four states' design teams, in rural and urban design teams, and large and small design teams) and (b) across design team members (i.e., within family experts, middle managers, front-line practitioners, non-child welfare professionals, university faculty facilitators, etc.).

SIMILAR FINDINGS USING DIFFERENT INTERVENTIONS

The outcomes associated with the design teams were surprisingly similar across each site and state. Despite cross-state and -site uniqueness, this finding nevertheless may be predictable. All sites relied on a learning systems represented by the design team process (Lawson, 2000; Lawson, Petersen, & Briar-Lawson, 2001). Structuring comparable and identical teams, while making efforts to create enabling, safe, and secure settings, may alone account for the similarities. Moreover, several sites relied on Nancy Petersen's pioneering work with the design team process. Other facilitators adopted components in her learning progression, and they used some of her action learning tools and exercises. Furthermore, many of the sites shared ideas and learned from each other throughout the design team process.

These similarities cannot be allowed to gloss over many differences. Some stemmed from contextual circumstances associated with each design team. State specific differences also impacted implementation. For instance, some design teams were located in states in which state agencies have considerable power and authority. In contrast, Colorado offers a county-based system. Furthermore, some states had close partnerships with universities; others were not as strong.

Site-specific differences also affected implementation, including differences related to location in rural or urban communities; the presence, or absence, of pre-existing community collaborations; and the willingness of key agencies to participate in the design team process. Last, but not least, faculty facilitators displayed different levels of commitment to the design team process. At least two facilitators did not implement the design team process as it was originally planned (Lawson, 2000). Consistent with Wenger's (1999) observation that it is impossible to control and manipulate learning outcomes, it also is impossible to control and manipulate faculty facilitators (Lawson, 2000). When cookie-cutter approaches to training are required, along with precise implementation protocols that safeguard fidelity, design-team like learning systems may not be the best alternative for learning and competency development.

Even so, different design teams, operating in diverse contexts, produce identical, similar, and comparable outcomes. This important and interesting finding needs to be interpreted, albeit briefly.

From Social Learning Theory to Sociocultural Learning Theory

Design teams for learning are intended to result in collaborative working teams in practice. The implication is that the team, i.e., a group of people, is the key unit of engagement and analysis. In contrast, most learning theory, including social learning theory, and the vast majority of training approaches target individuals, and they stop at the level of the individual (e.g., Rogoff, 1998).

As indicated earlier in this analysis, emergent sociocultural learning theory responds to needs for a complex theory of learning and development. It focuses on groups (teams), including how their participation in joint activities (e.g., collaborative practices) may be transformed. *Cognition and learning, in this perspective, are not merely individual properties; they also belong to a group or team.* In other words, the design team is a cognitive community (Dillenbourg, 1999), and, in this team setting, cognition is itself a collaborative process (e.g., Rogoff, 1998). According to Rogoff (1998):

> . . . collaboration is a process that can take many forms, whether intended or accidental, mutual or one-sided, face-to-face, shoulder-to-shoulder, or distant, congenial or contested: *the key feature is that in collaboration people are involved in other people's thinking processes through shared endeavors.* (Rogoff, 1998, p. 728, emphasis added)

Apparently, the design teams in this study promoted shared thinking; and shared thinking yielded identical, similar, and comparable outcomes across the four states. While at any given point in time, cognition and learning may be unevenly distributed among design team members, over time members report similar and identical changes in their commitments, practices, and, by implication, their professional identities (see also Wenger, 1999). Shared thinking and outcomes were fostered by an important combination of team composition, including family experts, and skillful facilitation, including the creation of safe, secure, and empowering social and institutional settings.

These reported changes in both individuals and groups are important because some sociocultural theorists recommend against research and evaluation protocols that require conventional pre- and post-training designs and analysis of variance statistical analyses (e.g., Rogoff, 1998). This evaluation presents an alternative possibility (see also Wenger, 1999). Specifically, a focus on the team (group) need not occur at the expense of a simultaneous focus on individual learning and development. In brief, it appears that individual learning and social learning are not antithetical to sociocultural theories of learning. Of course, this observation must be couched against the methodological limits of this evaluation, including the requirements of the grants that supported it.

Here, it is important to report that the desired outcomes and evaluation requirements of the grants supporting this initiative provided a structure that both enabled and constrained the design team process and its evaluation. The original request for proposals for the grants, like their reporting formats and requirements, were structured by training and competency-related discourse. This training discourse, with its focus on individuals, trainers, training protocols and curriculum, and competencies, was a significant constraint to the work reported here. To reiterate, the design team process operates from learning systems approach, and it relies on different discourses. Operating within a learning systems approach, but having to evaluate, report back, and use the training discourse constrained innovation. These constraints were more powerful because the majority of the faculty facilitators and other participants knew only the discourse and practices of training. Learning related discourses involving the design teams and the design team model were new to nearly everyone.

Paradoxically, constraining features and forces often materialize as enabling new opportunities and understanding. The reporting and evaluation requirements for the grant were perceived and experienced by many members of the initiative as constraints. These requirements compelled a focus on individual learning and development and competencies. If this initiative had been allowed to operate free of these grant-requirements, the evaluation might have looked very different. Specifically, it might not have attended to individual learning and development. Instead, it would have focused on teams and settings.

In short, if the evaluation had been oriented in this way, the important finding that it yielded–namely, that the design team process yields both individual learning and development as well as group learning and systems change–would have been lost. This is a serendipitous finding about both the evaluation and the design team process.

The Generativity of Learning Systems

While training systems are stability- and certainty-oriented, design teams as learning systems are vehicles for innovation. While training is oriented toward dissemination and reproduction of existing knowledge, skill, and understanding, learning systems have generative capacities. Design teams generate new knowledge, skills, competencies and understanding as they design new service delivery strategies and systems (Lawson, under review).

In accordance with the original plan for their operation, design teams had three related effects (Lawson, under review). Some had *multiplier effects*–i.e., one innovation led to another inside each team. Some had *contagion effects*–i.e., some design team members gave to non-members in their own agencies and in other agencies new knowledge, practices, and competencies. And three teams (Colorado, Utah, and Nevada) had *ripple effects*–i.e., some design teams helped catalyze changes in policy and in inter-agency relations at the state level. These multiple benefits are difficult to track and control. In contrast to training systems with their often-contrived attempts to control, track, and manipulate, learning systems like these design teams yield unpredictable, uncontrollable, and yet high desirable changes such as these benefits (Wenger, 1999).

Lingering Questions

At this point, the design teams are somewhat like black boxes. They are alike in that all are black boxes, and it remains intriguing and important that they yield identical, comparable, and similar outcomes. The fact remains, however, that these black box-like design teams are different, and each serves as a kind of container for processes that are not fully understood.

A suggested model for aspects of the micro-dynamics of design teams has been presented elsewhere (Lawson, Petersen, & Briar-Lawson, 2001). This model may guide aspects of future evaluations and research into the design team process. However, more methodological work is required. For example, process evaluations and more sensitive methods are needed to identify, describe, and explain the design team dynamics.

LIMITATIONS

This initiative and the design team process are complex changes. Evaluation designs are still being developed in response to the requirements and characteristics of these kinds of initiatives (e.g., Connell, Kubisch et al., 1997; Lawson, 1999). This evaluation must be framed against the new challenges for evaluators. The meta-evaluation findings, which are not reported here, may be as important as the findings about the initiative and the design team process.

This evaluation relied on self-reports. While self-reports are informative, they do not substitute for observational data. The next phase in this evaluation, had the grant continued, would have been observational studies sensitive to changes in practice and in systems.

Study participants noted that they learned a lot, shared information, collaborated more, and valued the experience. They also gave specific examples of changes that happened in service delivery in response to design team conversations.

On the other hand, this evaluation did not examine changes over time. In the present study, participants described benefits associated with the design teams retroactively. Little is known related to whether the design team actually created enhanced practice, collaboration, service integration, personal growth, etc. Furthermore, it is less clear whether families have benefited from these changes in practice and policy.

Identifying and measuring these two important variables (i.e., changes in practice and policy; and the attendant benefits for families) over time is difficult, even daunting. Future evaluation strategies need to explore the impacts of design teams and their contagion effects on everyday practice and agency effectiveness. These evaluations should not be limited to self-report.

CONCLUSIONS

Design teams are empowering learning and action systems. They convene professionals and past recipients of services to redesign child welfare practice and related services so they are more responsive to the multiple needs of families. Design teams in this study are effective and successful. They work as planned.

In this study, design teams members in Utah, Colorado, Nevada, and New Mexico indicated that there were many outcomes that resulted from the design team process. Design teams:

   a. promoted family-centered practice and interprofessional collaboration;
   b. enhanced service delivery by educating service providers about core competencies and increasing collaboration and service integration to meet co-occurring needs;
   c. fostered personal growth and self-awareness among design team participants, especially the family experts that served on them; and
   d. supported workers who felt under-appreciated and lonely.

In light of the data presented here, the original questions can be addressed anew. Can child welfare systems respond to new policy changes? Have professionals working in child welfare responded favorably to the transition from AFDC to TANF? Can social and health service providers learn to understand, assess, and address the co-occurring needs of the most vulnerable families? Can professionals learn to collaborate with each other and with families? The data here suggest that they can.

Design teams in Utah, Colorado, Nevada, and New Mexico were able to successfully provide learning, training, and capacity-building assistance to child welfare and its companion systems. Multiple forms of collaboration involving professionals, agencies, universities, families, and entire neighborhood communities were developed. New practices that emphasized the co-occurrence of needs and family-centered and interprofessional collaboration were formed. Practices and policies related to enhanced service integration and reduced duplication were created. Personal growth, knowledge generation, and mutual support were fostered, albeit indirectly.

Design teams are continuing to meet and interact. As they do, their "curriculum" continues to develop. In addition to the impacts presented in this study, others no doubt will follow as the design team's intended contagion effects continue. Systems change and cross-systems change are facilitated in the process.

NOTES

1. The Children's Bureau is not responsible for the interpretations and views presented in this paper.
2. Nancy Petersen, University of Nevada-Reno, is the primary author of this mission statement.
3. For a quick review of this literature, see Lawson, Petersen, and Briar-Lawson (2001). The more extensive review is provided in Lawson, Briar-Lawson et al. (1999).
4. See Lawson, Anderson-Butcher et al. (in press) to review evaluation data related to the key components of effective design team processes.
5. Although the case can be made that family-centered practice is not the same as family-centered collaboration, design team members apparently treated them as synonyms. We return to this finding in the discussion.

REFERENCES

Argyris, C. (1996). Actionable knowledge: Design causality in the service of consequential theory. *Journal of Applied Behavioral Science, 32,* 390-406.

Argryis, C., & Schön, D. (1996). *Theory in practice: Increasing professional effectiveness II.* Reading, MA: Addison-Wesley.

Beresford, P. (2000). Service user's knowledges and social work theory: Conflict or collaboration? *British Journal of Social Work,* 30, 489-503.

Berns, D., & Drake, B. (1999). Combining child welfare and welfare reform at a local level: Policy and practice. *Journal of the American Public Health Services Association,* 57 (1), 26-34.

Briar-Lawson, K. (1998). Capacity-building for family-centered services and supports. *Social Work, 43,* 539-550.

Briar-Lawson, K. (2001). Integrating employment, economic supports, and family capacity-building. In A. Sallee, H. Lawson, & K. Briar-Lawson (Eds.), *Innovative practices with vulnerable children and families* (pp.13-32). Dubuque, IA: Eddie Bowers Publishers, Inc.

Briar-Lawson, K., Lawson, H., Petersen, N., Harris, N., Sallee, A., Hoffman, T., & Derezotes, D. (1999, January). Meeting the co-occurring needs of child welfare families through collaboration. Paper presented at the Society for Social Work Research, Austin, TX.

Cole, M. (1997). Cultural mechanisms of cognitive development. In E. Amsel & K. Renninger (Eds.), *Change and development: Issues of theory, method, and application* (pp. 245-264). Mawah, NJ: Lawrence Erlbaum Associates.

Connell, J., Kubish, A., Schorr, L., & Weiss, C. (Eds.) (1995). *New approaches to evaluating community initiatives: Concepts, methods and contexts.* Washington, DC: The Aspen Institute.

Derr, M. & Taylor, M. J. (1999). *The link between childhood and adult abuse among long term welfare recipients.* Unpublished paper. Social Research Institute of the Graduate School of Social Work, University of Utah, Salt Lake City, UT.

Dillenbourg, P. (1999). Introduction: What do you mean by "collaborative learning"? In P. Dillenbourg (Ed.), *Collaborative learning: Cognitive and computational approaches* (pp. 1-19). Amsterdam & New York: Pergamon.

Gee, J., & Green, J. (1998). Discourse analysis, learning and social practice: A methodological study. In P. Pearson & A. Iran-Nejad (Eds.), *Review of research in education 23* (pp. 119-170). Washington, DC: American Educational Research Association.

Kessler, R., Nelson, C., McGonagle, K., Edlund, M., Frank, R., & Leaf, P. (1996). The epidemiology of co-occurring addictive and mental disorders: Implications for prevention and service utilization. *American Journal of Orthopsychiatry, 66,* 17-31.

Kessler, R., Gillis-Light, J., Magee, W., Kendler, K., & Eaves, L. (1997). Childhood adversity and adult psychopathology. In I. Gotlib & B. Wheaton (Eds.), *Stress and adversity over the life course: Trajectories and turning points* (pp. 29-49). New York & Cambridge: Cambridge University Press.

Lawson, H. (1998). Academically-based community scholarship, consultation as collaborative problem-solving, and a collective-responsibility model for the helping fields. *Journal of Educational and Psychological Consultation, 9,* 195-232.

Lawson, H. (1999). Journey analysis: A framework for integrating consultation and evaluation in complex change initiatives. *Journal of Educational and Psychological Consultation, 10,* 145-172.

Lawson, H. (2000, September). Training systems, learning systems, and the challenges of intervention and evaluation. Paper presented at the National Child Welfare Conference: New Century Innovations for Vulnerable Children, Youth, and Families. Snowbird, UT.

Lawson, H. (2001). Back to the future: New century professionalism and collaborative leadership for comprehensive, community-based systems of care. In A. Sallee, H. Lawson, & K. Briar-Lawson (Eds.), *Innovative practices with vulnerable children and families* (pp. 393-419). Dubuque, IA: Eddie Bowers Publishers, Inc.

Lawson, H. (under review). Training systems, learning systems, and the challenges of collaboration. Manuscript submitted for publication.

Lawson, H., Anderson-Butcher, D., Petersen, N., & Barkdull, C. (in press). Design teams as learning systems for complex systems change: Evaluation data and implications for higher education. *Journal of Health & Social Policy.*

Lawson, H. A., & Barkdull, C. (2001). Gaining the collaborative advantage and promoting systems and cross-systems change. In A. Sallee, K. Briar-Lawson, & H. A. Lawson (Eds.), *New century practice with child welfare families* (pp. 245-270). Dubuque, IA: Eddie Bowers Publishers Inc.

Lawson, H., Briar-Lawson, K. Petersen, N., Harris, N., Sallee, A., Hoffman, T., & Derezotes, D. (1999, April). The development of an empowerment-oriented model for interprofessional collaboration, organizational improvement, and policy change. Paper presented at the American Educational Research Association, Montreal, Quebec, Canada.

Lawson, H., Khaja, K., & Soto, E. (1999). *Launching a journey analysis of the El Paso County Department of Human Services.* Salt Lake City, UT: Institute for Social Research, Graduate School of Social Work, University of Utah.

Lawson, H., Petersen, N., & Briar-Lawson K. (2001). From conventional training to empowering design teams for collaboration and systems change. In A. Sallee, K. Briar-Lawson, & H. A. Lawson (Eds.), *New century practice with child welfare families* (pp. 361-392). Dubuque, IA: Eddie Bowers Publishers Inc.

Lawson, H., & Sailor, W. (2000). Integrating services, collaborating, and developing connections with schools. *Focus on Exceptional Children, 33* (2), 1-22.

Lincoln, Y. S., & Guba, E. G. (1985). *Naturalistic inquiry.* Beverly Hills. Sage.

Miles, M. B., & Huberman, A. M. (1994). *Qualitative data analyses.* Newbury Park, CA: Sage.

Nespor, J. (1994). *Knowledge in motion: Space, time and the curriculum in undergraduate physics and management.* Philadelphia: Taylor & Francis.

Patton, M. Q. (1990). *Qualitative evaluation and research methods.* Newbury Park, CA: Sage.

Rogoff, B. (1998). Cognition as collaborative process. In D. Kuhn & R. Siegler (Eds.), *Handbook of child psychology, Volume 2* (pp. 679-744). New York: John Wiley & Sons.

Rogoff, B., Matusov, E., & White, C. (1996). Models of teaching and learning: Participation in a community of learners. In D. Olson & N. Torrance (Eds.), *The handbook of education and human development: New models of teaching, learning, and schooling* (pp. 388-414). Oxford, UK: Blackwell.

Salomon, G., & Perkins, D. (1998). Individual and social aspects of learning. In P. Pearson & A. Iran-Nejad (Eds.), *Review of research in education 23* (pp. 1-24). Washington, DC: American Educational Research Association.

U.S. Department of Human Services. (1999). *Blending perspectives and building common ground: A report to congress on substance abuse and child protection.* Washington, DC: U.S. Government Printing Office.

VanWagoner, P., Boyer, R., Wiesen, M., DeNiro-Ashton, D., & Lawson, H. A. (2001). Introducing child welfare neighborhood teams that promote collaboration and community-based systems of care. In A. Sallee, K. Briar-Lawson, & H. A. Lawson (Eds.), *New century practice with child welfare families* (pp. 323-360). Dubuque, IA: Eddie Bowers Publishers Inc.

Vygotsky, L. S. (1978). *Mind in society.* Cambridge, MA: Harvard University Press.

Wenger, E. (1999). *Communities of practice: Learning, meaning, and identity.* London & New York: Cambridge University Press.

Examination of Racial Imbalance for Children in Foster Care: Implications for Training

Kathleen Belanger, MSSW

SUMMARY. Concerned with the high number of African American children in out-of-home care in an East Texas county, the regional administrator of a state public child welfare agency asked its IV-E partnered university to examine the kinds of training the agency might need to address the problem. A semi-annual time-series model from January 1997 to June 1999 was constructed to track the proportion of African American children at three critical case junctures: investigation, case opening, and removal of the child to out-of-home care. In addition, the study analyzed characteristics of the county's population, including racial changes and poverty. The study found that African American children were referred to public child welfare at twice the rate of Anglo children, with the ratio increasing during case progression. The study also found a higher proportion of African American children in the community and a higher poverty rate, particularly for African American children, than what was previously understood. The study not only provided details of racial distribution over time and over case disposition, but also highlighted the importance of understanding problems within a community and organizational context. The study further suggests that training include generalist and advanced generalist social work education, con-

---

Kathleen Belanger is Director of the Child Welfare Professional Development Project, School of Social Work, Stephen F. Austin State University, P. O. Box 6104 SFA Station, Nacogdoches, TX 75961 (E-mail: kbelanger@sfasu.edu).

[Haworth co-indexing entry note]: "Examination of Racial Imbalance for Children in Foster Care: Implications for Training." Belanger, Kathleen. Co-published simultaneously in *Journal of Health & Social Policy* (The Haworth Press, Inc.) Vol. 15, No. 3/4, 2002, pp. 163-176; and: *Evaluation Research in Child Welfare: Improving Outcomes Through University-Public Agency Partnerships* (ed: Katharine Briar-Lawson, and Joan Levy Zlotnik) The Haworth Press, Inc., 2002, pp. 163-176. Single or multiple copies of this article are available for a fee from The Haworth Document Delivery Service [1-800-HAWORTH, 9:00 a.m. - 5:00 p.m. (EST). E-mail address: getinfo@haworthpressinc.com].

sidering practice with systems of all sizes, to assess, prevent, treat and evaluate interventions designed for the safety, permanency and well-being of children. *[Article copies available for a fee from The Haworth Document Delivery Service: 1-800-HAWORTH. E-mail address: <getinfo@haworthpressinc.com> Website: <http://www.HaworthPress.com> © 2002 by The Haworth Press, Inc. All rights reserved.]*

KEYWORDS. Child welfare, poverty, foster care, African American children, social work education, Title IV-E, permanency, university collaboration

INTRODUCTION

In one East Texas county, 50% of the children entering foster care are African American. This region of the Texas Department of Protective and Regulatory Services (TDPRS) has a productive and active IV-E partnership that includes preparation of students to enter public child welfare, staff assistance in obtaining social work degrees, pre-service and in-service training, and training for foster parents. The region's administration, therefore, requested that the university examine the issue and make recommendations, particularly relating to staff training.

Literature Review

The high proportion of African American children in the child welfare system has long been recognized as a national reality, comprising 40-50% of the foster care population (Garland et al., 1998). Multiple factors are attributed to this over-representation, including poverty, institutional discrimination and worker bias (Hollingsworth, 1998). In addition, children in kinship care are counted in foster care statistics; since African Americans tend to use kinship homes more frequently, some view their inclusion in foster care statistics as an overrepresentation (Hollingsworth, 1998). Low family income is considered the strongest indicator of removal of a child; additionally, the subsequent loss of services and income assistance further reduces a family's chances for reunification (Lindsey, 1991). In analyzing census statistics, The Children's Defense Fund states that African American children are more than three times as likely to live in poverty than Anglo children (Sherman, 1994). Corcoran and Chaudry (1997) point to the relationship between poverty and race, noting "although White children constituted 60% of all children who were poor in 1992, almost 90% of the long-term poor children were African American" (p. 47). Everett, Chipungu, and Leashore (1997) state that the majority of reports to TDPRS for African American children are for "alleged neglect" (p. 184). The authors further state child neglect is "ignored by society" and is described as "the most forgotten form of maltreatment and the most frequent reason for placement." Its prevalence tends to be associated with "low-income, large, and multi-problem families and with families of color" (Everett et al., p. 184).

Moreover, the co-occurrence of poverty and parental substance abuse are cause for increasing concern. In both client level and macro-level studies, substance abuse associated with poverty is directly linked with child maltreatment (Albert et al., 2000; Murphy et al., 1991; Garbarino and Kostelny, 1992; GAO, 1997). In presenting a history of and forecast for public child welfare, Schorr deplores the "deepening poverty and severe family and social problems that add to caseloads" while calling for social work professionals in the child welfare system to form partnerships and engage communities in solving the root problems such as poverty (Schorr, 2000).

The purpose of this study was to determine the extent of the overrepresentation of African American children in care in this specific county, explore possible relationships with other factors and posit further areas for investigation or training. The study, therefore, addressed the following eight issues:

- What specifically is the ratio of African American children in foster care? Do the proportions reflect the proportions of African American children in the population?
- If there is a disproportionate number relative to the population, is this a relatively new phenomenon, or has it existed in previous years?
- At which point does the ratio of African American children in care become disproportionate to population statistics?
- Are there more initial complaints filed proportionately for African American families?
- Is there a greater proportion of validated complaints?
- Does the ratio of African American children increase or decrease with placement in out-of-home care?
- Are there case-specific factors such as allegation, age of child, and family problems that differ by race?
- Are there non-case-specific factors that could be related to the ratio of African American children in the county's foster care system?

METHODOLOGY

The region was aware that 50% of the children entering foster care were African American (compared with an African American county population of 31%), and that African American children in the county took longer to achieve permanency than their Anglo American counterparts. However, it was unclear at which point overrepresentation relative to the population occurs. For example, if all children referred to TDPRS are of a single race or ethnicity, then only those children will ever be in out-of-home care. We, therefore, chose a semi-annual time-series model to determine the actual racial proportions. We worked directly with the agency's management information system (MIS) staff to obtain de-identified data for six-month intervals from January 1997 to June 1999. The de-identified data was then further examined to answer the questions above. However, there were several difficulties. First of all, the MIS system appeared better able to provide in-depth tracking of specific cases rather than allow for aggregating data into usable information.

In addition, there were numerous and sometimes confusing (to the worker) codes for each case action. We worked directly with staff to assure that this report was based on the best judgments possible concerning use of codes and inferences to be made from them. In addition, the study tracked racial proportions for all cases at three critical case junctures: investigation, case opening, and removal of the child to out-of-home care. The study also examined the specific allegations of lack of supervision, physical abuse, sexual abuse and abandonment to determine whether they were also racially disproportionate. Finally, the study analyzed characteristics of the organization and of the county's entire population, including changing ethnicity and poverty.

RESULTS

Phase I: Examination of Racial Distribution at Critical Case Junctures

A. Investigation

While African Americans account for 30% of the county's population, African American children account for 39% of the child population, and 50-58% of the referrals for investigations for abuse or neglect. To examine the ratios more accurately, the number of children referred to the system was determined relative to the total child population, providing the number of children by ethnicity per 1000 children in the county. As shown in Table 1, African American children are twice as likely to be referred to TDPRS for investigation (37 per 1000 children for African Americans in 1/97 compared with 17 per 1000 children for Anglos).

In other words, overrepresentation begins with the complaint. As also shown in Table 1, the overrepresentation is not a recent phenomenon, and in fact was reduced somewhat during the last year of the study. The factors influ-

TABLE 1. Comparison of Children by Ethnicity: CPS Investigations from 1997 Through June 16, 1999 and 1990 U.S. Census Data

	1990 U.S. CENSUS	1997 JAN. CPS	Per 1000 Child Pop.	1997 JULY CPS	Per 1000 Child Pop.	1998 JAN. CPS	Per 1000 Child Pop.	1998 JULY CPS	Per 1000 Child Pop.	1999 JAN. CPS	Per 1000 Child Pop.
Total Pop. (18 yr. and under)	67,960	1,841		2,051		2,024		1,815		1,754	
Anglo	52.6 35,747	33.0 610	17	29.8 611	17	30.4 615	17	36.1 655	18	36.3 636	18
African American	38.7 26,348	52.9 979	37	57.7 1,183	44	55.4 1,121	43	50.3 913	35	50.6 851	32

Source: 1990 U.S. Census Data, TDPRS CAPS Data

encing a higher referral rate at system entry have existed for at least two years, and probably longer. However, it does appear that since the beginning of 1998 both the total number of referrals and the proportion of African American referrals is diminishing, with 32 per 1000 African American children referred compared with 18 per 1000 Anglo children (see Figure 1).

B. Case Opening

Not only are African American children referred to the public child welfare system at a higher rate (approximately 2:1 relative to the population), but the ratio of cases that were opened (reason to believe) is 3:1 and 4:1 for African American children compared with Anglo children, widening the disparity further. The higher rate of case validation continues over time, even to the present (see Table 2).

C. Removal of the Child to Out-Of-Home Care

We used the reason for closure of the investigation "removal/substitute care" as the best indicator available for comparing racial differences in placement into out-of-home care. The proportion of investigations terminating in out-of-home care is consistently higher for African-American children. Controlling for the population, African American children are placed in out-of-home care at 3 to 17 times the rate of Anglo American children, depending on the time period (see Table 3).

In other words, out-of-home care is the relative disposition of 3-5% of African American children's cases, compared with 1-2% of Anglo children's cases, widening the disparity even further.

FIGURE 1. Ethnicity Comparison of CPS Investigations: 1997-June 16, 1999

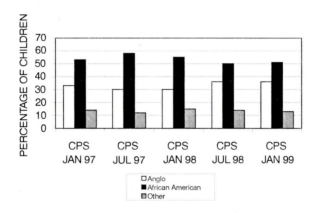

Source: TDPRS CAPS Data

TABLE 2. Validated Intakes

	1-97-7-97 % valid	Per 1000 Child Pop.	7-97-12-97 % valid	Per 1000 Child Pop.	1-98-7-98 % valid	Per 1000 Child Pop.	7-98-12-98 % valid	Per 1000 Child Pop.	1-99-6-15-99 % valid	Per 1000 Child Pop.
African American	33.2	12	36.2	16	39.3	17	35.2	12	19.4	6
Anglo	23.6	4	25.0	4	28.5	5	27.5	5	12.0	2

Source: 1990 U.S. Census Data, TDPRS CAPS Data (Overall Disposition = reason to believe: RTB)

TABLE 3. Percent and Number of Investigations Ending in Removal by Ethnicity

	1-97-7-97 % in sub care	Per 1000 Child Pop.	7-97-12-97 % in sub care	Per 1000 Child Pop.	1-98-7-98 % in sub care	Per 1000 Child Pop.	7-98-12-98 % in sub care	Per 1000 Child Pop.	1-99-6-15-99 % in sub care	Per 1000 Child Pop.
African American	3.0 n = 29	1.1	4.6 n = 54	2	5 n = 59	2.2	4.4 n = 40	1.5	5.4 n = 46	1.7
Anglo	2.5 n = 15	0.4	2.5 n = 15	0.4	2.3 n = 14	0.3	1.8 n = 12	0.3	0.8 n = 5	0.1

Source: 1990 U.S. Census Data, TDPRS CAPS Data (Reason for Closure-Removal/Substitute Care)

The number of African American children per 1000 child population, compared with the number of Anglo children is depicted for each of the three critical case junctures in Figure 2.

Phase II: Racial Distribution Relative to Allegation and Child's Age

A. Allegations

We explored several factors to determine whether there were any substantive differences in the case depending upon the child's race. Four of the more serious allegations were examined: lack of supervision, physical abuse, sexual abuse and abandonment. No conclusions could be drawn from the data because of fluctuations and small numbers of cases in certain categories compounded by the fact that one family alone could account for several cases in any category.

B. Age of Child Referred

Table 4 shows the age of the children in out-of-home care on June 1, 1999 (the most current data available at the time). One-third of all the children in

FIGURE 2. Comparative Ethnicity of Children from Investigation to Substitute Care

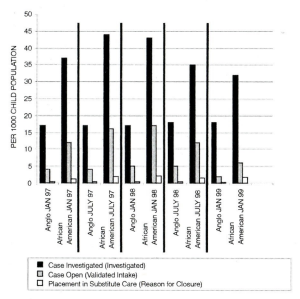

Source: 1990 U.S. Census Data, TDPRS CAPS Data

out-of-home care (56 of 169) in the county were African American infants. In addition, while the numbers of African American children in care decline as the age of the child increases, 79% of all Anglo children in care are either infants or teenagers, with teenagers representing the largest Anglo grouping (45%).

Phase III: Examination of County: Child Population, Poverty, Kinship Care, and Organizational Cultural Competence

In order to put the findings in context, we examined the county for several factors relevant to child welfare.

A. County Population

According to the 1990 U. S. Census, the population of the county included 239,397 persons, with approximately 64% Anglo (Non-Hispanic), 31% African American (Non-Hispanic), and 8% Asian, Hispanic, American Indian and "Other." However, the child population (18 years and under for the purposes of this report) was 67,960, of which only 53% were Anglo and 39% African American. Using child population data dramatically alters the base proportions used for comparisons (see Figure 3).

In fact, this county has the third highest percentage of African American children in the state (Kids Count, 1997).

B. Poverty

This East Texas county is very poor, with poverty much higher among African American families. According to the U. S. Census (1995), 31% of the children in the county live in poverty compared with only 22% nationally. In addition, 64% of the families with children in poverty in this county are African American (Figure 4).

TABLE 4. Children in Substitute Care on June 1, 1999, by Age

AGE	0 to 3	4 to 6	7 to 11	12 and over	Total
African American	56(43%)	28(22%)	25(19%)	21(16%)	130
Anglo	13(34%)	5(13%)	3(8%)	17(45%)	39

Source: TDPRS CAPS Data

FIGURE 3. Ethnicity Comparison of 1990 U.S. Census Data: Total Population
to Child Population

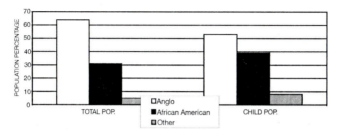

Source: 1990 U.S. Census Data

C. Kinship Care

Kinship care has been an important out-of-home placement in this county, particularly for African American children, possibly inflating the numbers of African American children in out-of-home temporary care when in reality their care is intended to be permanent and an extension of home.

D. Organizational Cultural Competence

The county's staff is racially diverse, with 50% of the direct service and administrative staff ethnic or racial minorities (42% African American). In addition, direct service and administrative staff receives comprehensive training in cultural competence at least every two years as part of a statewide training initiative. While this does not assure cultural competence, the data does not preclude it either.

DISCUSSION

The study did find that African American children enter the TDPRS system in this county and are eventually placed in out-of-home care at rates disproportionately higher than their Anglo American counterparts. However, the study also found environmental factors that are directly linked in the literature to participation in the child welfare system.

The Role of Environmental Factors

There is a great deal of research that points to level of income of the parent, rather than maltreatment, as a more significant indicator of whether or not the child will be placed in out-of-home care. Pecora, Whittaker, and Maluccio

FIGURE 4. Ethnicity Comparison: Families Below the Poverty Level in 1989 with Children Under 18 Years

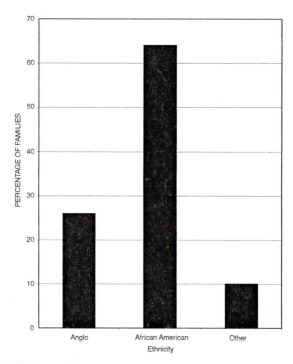

Source: 1990 U.S. Census Data

(1992) state "many advocates would argue that a significant number of children would be prevented from being placed if sufficient resources were available for family income assistance, housing, health care, and crisis intervention support" (p. 27). He further adds while there has been an increase in "real need on the part of families and children," there has also been "almost two decades of steady erosion in program funding" (Pecora et al., 1992, p. 27).

Because this particular county has been identified as having a very high poverty rate, the third highest proportion of African American children in the state, with sixty-four percent of the families with children in poverty African American, the higher poverty rates alone may explain racial imbalances in the child welfare system. In fact, the proportion of African American children vs. Anglo children in foster care in this county (2:1) directly mirrors the proportion of African American poor children vs. Anglo children in this county (2:1).

The state does not have income data available for families in its child welfare system; therefore, we could perform no analyses directly relating case outcome to family poverty. However, the findings raise several questions. Does poverty, at least in some cases, cause entry into public child welfare? If so why? Does racial discrimination in the workforce result not only in inadequate family income, but the family's inability to care for its children? Are there factors directly related to obtaining and maintaining employment/income (lack of education or skills, mental illness or substance abuse, etc.) that also relate to child abuse and neglect? Are there factors that determine both poverty and entry into child welfare: racial discrimination within multiple community organizations and systems, judicial and institutional definitions that are culturally and/or racially biased, etc.? Inclusion of data related to family income in state management information systems could provide much clearer and relatively low cost answers to some of these issues, and make further research into other causal or relational factors possible.

In addition, the majority of children in kinship care in the United States are African American (Scannapieco & Jackson, 1996, p.194). Many, therefore, contend that foster care statistics, by including kinship care, over-represent African American families (Hollingsworth, 1998). The administration verifies that there are substantial numbers of children placed in kinship care in this particular county that may account for at least some of the racial imbalance in out-of-home care.

Institutional Discrimination/Worker Bias

The literature cites several known problems that could be a result of institutional racism and discrimination at worst, and lack of cultural competence at best (Gold, 1997; Dillon, 1994).

The child welfare staff in this county is racially diverse and has received training in cultural competence at varying levels over time. While we could not conclude that the staff was indeed culturally competent without a deeper examination of specific casework, it would be a mistake to conclude that the public child welfare agency is discriminatory. Even if there is institutional discrimination in this county, it may very well exist in other agencies or systems, resulting greater family stress, fewer services offered to prevent family problems and higher referrals to public child welfare.

IMPLICATIONS FOR TRAINING

Child welfare training is often envisioned as delivering a set of knowledge, values and skills that enable staff members to develop certain competencies for work with individual children and families to achieve successful case outcomes. However, many of the problems faced by the child welfare system and its staff are problems with larger systems, with groups, organizations and communities. The powerful relationship between poverty and child maltreatment (Sedlak and Broadhurst, 1996) suggests community wide strategies, forming alliances, advocacy, etc. (Courtney, 1999). Building on Barth's work in analyzing race and long-term foster care (Barth, 1997), Barth, Goodhand and Dickinson discuss in the 1999 Child Welfare Training Symposium the importance of community based child protection and the mechanisms to promote partnerships (p. 7). In addition, the symposium's action agenda includes in item 7 to assure that universities develop appropriate curricula for students, and pre-service and in-service training for child welfare practice. Specifically, "Participants recommended that universities . . . expand on the impact of poverty, health and mental health care availability, the impact of substance abuse, and the impact of family violence issues" (1999 Child Welfare Training Symposium, p. 129). Strategies to address the combination of issues involved in child maltreatment include provision of integrated service systems (Corrigan and Bishop, 1997), forming community partnerships (Waldfogel, 1997; GAO, 1997), cross-system training and collaboration (Tracy & Pine, 1997), including training in building collaborative relationships (GAO, 1997).

This study, intended as the initiation of development of cultural competence training, instead resulted in providing training for the regional administration and staff in understanding the larger contexts of child welfare work, particularly the issue of poverty as it relates to racial distributions in the child welfare system. Instead of spending further staff time and organizational resources in training that may not be warranted, the Title IV-E partnership redirected efforts to understanding root causes of ongoing difficulties in child welfare, and emphasized the need for well trained professionals competent in social work practice with systems of all sizes. Successful case outcomes may depend on the public child welfare worker's ability to assess problems, policies and legislation, design solutions, advocate for resources not just for one client or one caseload, but for the majority of children and families in the community who suffer from child maltreatment. This is not solely an administrative function. It is increasingly imperative for local child welfare staff to demonstrate leadership in identifying problems, to develop partnerships and collaborations, to create and implement change and secure resources sorely lacking in many of the communities. It takes a skilled workforce, from front-line staff to administration, who understand families in their environment, in their communities, willing and capable of planning and implementing change in systems of all sizes. In addition, further research into these issues is mandatory, not just for adequate staff training, but for structuring of the workforce and deploying resources. This is the precise focus of generalist and advanced generalist social work education provided by accredited social work programs.

Title IV-E partnerships, by their very nature expand the understanding of the role of larger systems, build collaborations, and link students trained in generalist practice to public child welfare agencies sorely in need of a workforce with this background. By examining, from a generalist perspective, the issue of the overrepresentation of African American children in out-of-home care in one East Texas county care, this study emphasizes the benefits of university/agency partnerships. University/agency collaboration can more readily explore complex issues in child welfare practice. Through such collaborations, Title IV-E training funds can be used more efficiently, analyzing true training needs, providing curricula and training in those areas, and targeting further need for research for the numerous important but unanswered questions. University/agency partnerships further emphasize the need for all members of the child welfare community to understand problems within a broader context so that we can achieve the outcomes of permanency, safety and well-being for children.

REFERENCES

Albert, V., Klein, D., Noble, A., Zahand, E., & Holtby, S. (2000). Identifying substance abusing delivering women: Consequences for child maltreatment reports. *Child Abuse & Neglect: The International Journal, 24* (2), 173-183.

Barth, R. P., Goodhand, J., & Dickinson, N. S. (1999). Reconciling competing values in the delivery of child welfare services under ASFA, MEPA, and community-based child protection. *Monograph of 1999 Child Welfare Training Symposium.*

Belanger, K. (1996). *Needs assessment for Deep East Texas.* Unpublished manuscript. Stephen F. Austin State University.

Child Welfare League of America. (1993). *Cultural Competence Self-Assessment Instrument.* Washington, DC: CWLA.

Corcoran, M. E., & Chaudry, A. (1997). The dynamics of childhood poverty. *The Future of Children, 7* (2), 40-54.

Dillon, D. (1994). Understanding and assessment of intragroup dynamics in family foster care: African American families. *Child Welfare, 73* (2), 129-139.

Duncan, D. F. (1998). Prevention issues: Some cautionary notes. In R. L. Hampton, V. Senatore, & T. P. Gullotta (Eds.), *Substance abuse, family violence, and child welfare* (pp. 249-262). Thousand Oaks: Sage Publications, Inc.

Everett, J., Chipungu, S., & Leashore, B. (Eds.). (1997). *Child Welfare: An Africentric perspective.* New Brunswick, NJ: Rutgers University Press.

Garbarino, J., & Kostelny, K. (1992). Child maltreatment as a community problem. *Child Abuse & Neglect, 16,* 455-464.

Garland, A., Ellis-MacLeod, E., Landsverk, J., Ganger, W., & Johnson, I. (1998). Minority populations in the child welfare system: The visibility hypothesis reexamined. *American Journal of Orthopsychiatry, 68* (1), 142-146.

Gould, K. (1997). Limiting damage is not enough: A minority perspective on child welfare issues. In Everett, J., Chipungu, S., & Leashore, B. (Eds.). (1997). *Child Welfare: An Africentric perspective.* New Brunswick, NJ: Rutgers University Press.

Hollingsworth, L. D. (1998). Promoting same-race adoption for children of color. *Social Work, 43* (2), 104-116.

Klein, D., Noble, A., Zahand, E., & Holtby, S. (2000). Identifying substance abusing delivering women: Consequences for child maltreatment reports. *Child Abuse & Neglect, 24* (2), 173-183.

Lindsey, D. (1991). Factors affecting the foster care placement decision: An analysis of national survey data. *American Journal of Orthopsychiatry, 61*(2), 272-281.

Murphy, J. M., Jellinek, M., Quinn, D., Smith, G., Poitrast, F., & Goshko, M. (1991). Substance abuse and serious child maltreatment: Prevelance, risk, and outcome in a court sample. *Child Abuse & Neglect, 15,* 197-211.

Onyskiw, J. E. & Harrison, M. J. (1999). Formative evaluation of a collaborative community-based child abuse prevention project. *Child Abuse & Neglect: The International Journal, 23* (11), 1069-1081.

Pecora, P., Whittaker, J., & Maluccio, A. (1992). *The child welfare challenge: Policy, practice, and research.* Hawthorne, NY: Aldine De Gruyter.

Scannapieco, M., & Jackson, S. (1996). Kinship care: The African American response to family preservation. *Social Work, 41* (2), 190-196.

Schorr, A. L. (2000). The bleak prospect for public child welfare. *Social Service Review, 74* (1), 124.

Sherman, A. (1994). *Wasting America's future: The Children's Defense Fund report on the costs of child poverty.* Boston: Beacon Press.

Texas Department of Protective and Regulatory Services. (2000). Child abuse and neglect fact sheet. Retrieved September 18, 2000 from the World Wide Web: www.tdprs.state.tx.us/Child_Protection/About_Child_Abuse/childfacts.aspmaltreatment reports.

Texas Kids Count Project. (1997). *African American children in Texas.* Austin: The Center for Public Policy Priorities.

Tracy, E. M. & Pine, B. A. (2000). Child welfare education and training: Future trends and influences. *Child Welfare, LXXIX* (1), 93-111.

United States Census Bureau. (1995). Model-based income and poverty estimates for Jefferson County, Texas in 1995. (www.census.gov/hhes/www/saipe/estimate/cty/cty48245.htm) (September 1, 1999).

U.S. Department of Health and Human Services. (1999). *1999 Child Welfare Training Symposium: Changing paradigms of child welfare practice: Responding to opportunities and challenges.* Administration for Children and Families, June, 1999.

United States General Accounting Office. (1997). *Child Protective Services: Complex challenges require new strategies* (GAO/HEHS-97-115). Washington, DC: GAO.

Waldfogel, J. (2000). Reforming child protective services. *Child Welfare, LXXIX* (1), 43-57.

Facing the Challenge of a Changing System: Training Child Welfare Workers in a Privatized Environment

Debora M. Ortega, MSW, PhD
Michelle M. Levy, MSW

SUMMARY. The state of Kansas' implementation of a privatized child welfare system is arguably an ambitious shift in child welfare service delivery. In an attempt to drastically improve services to vulnerable families, privatization resulted in intended and unintended consequences for the child welfare workforce. Some of these consequences, including the influx of inexperienced new workers, high worker turnover, and managing relationships with multiple partners, are issues that affect training needs of child welfare professionals. The following paper offers one approach to addressing these needs as well as identifying the challenges involved in training in a privatized environment. *[Article copies available for a fee from The Haworth Document Delivery Service: 1-800-HAWORTH. E-mail address: <getinfo@haworthpressinc.com> Website: <http://www.HaworthPress.com> © 2002 by The Haworth Press, Inc. All rights reserved.]*

KEYWORDS. Child welfare training, privatized child welfare services

---

Debora M. Ortega is Assistant Professor at the School of Social Welfare, University of Kansas. She is the Principal Investigator for the State of Kansas Private Provider Training Contract.

Michelle M. Levy is Child Welfare Program Coordinator at the School of Social Welfare, University of Kansas.

[Haworth co-indexing entry note]: "Facing the Challenge of a Changing System: Training Child Welfare Workers in a Privatized Environment." Ortega, Debora M., and Michelle M. Levy. Co-published simultaneously in *Journal of Health & Social Policy* (The Haworth Press, Inc.) Vol. 15, No. 3/4, 2002, pp. 177-187; and: *Evaluation Research in Child Welfare: Improving Outcomes Through University-Public Agency Partnerships* (ed: Katharine Briar-Lawson, and Joan Levy Zlotnik) The Haworth Press, Inc., 2002, pp. 177-187. Single or multiple copies of this article are available for a fee from The Haworth Document Delivery Service [1-800-HAWORTH, 9:00 a.m. - 5:00 p.m. (EST). E-mail address: getinfo@haworthpressinc.com].

177

INTRODUCTION

States and universities across the country are joined in collaborative partnerships to support the "reprofessionalization" of public sector child welfare. Through the Social Security Act Title IV-E and 462 funding, these partnerships enhance child welfare service delivery by improving the skills and knowledge of front-line workers. It has been demonstrated that professional education and training programs foster workers who are better prepared (Dhopper, Royse & Wolfe, 1990), more effective in service delivery (Olsen & Holmes, 1982; Albers, Reilly & Rittner, 1993) and less likely to leave public sector child welfare work (Child Welfare League of America, 1990).

Privatization and managed care principles are altering the nature of child welfare practice. One state's experience in adopting a privatized managed care system illustrates potential implications for the preparation and training of front-line child welfare workers in private agencies. The development of a strengths-based training curriculum highlighting the transfer of learning provides one example of "reprofessionalization" efforts within the private sector.

The Privatized Managed Care Service Model in Kansas

In 1997, Kansas became the first state in the country to fully privatize the major services of its child welfare system under a managed care model. This dramatic statewide change shifted responsibility for the delivery of family preservation, foster care and adoption services to private agencies. In this system, the Kansas Department of Social and Rehabilitation Services (SRS) continues to receive and investigate reports of alleged abuse and neglect. SRS then refers cases to contractors, provides ongoing case monitoring, and conducts most court actions. Private agency contractors are responsible for assessment, case planning and service provision in all family preservation, foster care and adoption cases. These services are provided either directly or through sub-contracts with other community-based agencies.

Impetus for Privatization

A convergence of the inadequacies in the child welfare system, a 1993 out-of-court settlement agreement with the American Civil Liberties Union, and renewed political and legal pressure for reform led to the dramatic privatization in Kansas. As in many states, escalating costs, poor performance and public misgivings plagued the Kansas child welfare system. The governor and state legislature publicly acknowledged the system's failings and called for restructuring (Kansas Action for Children, Inc., 1998). The privatized managed care service model emerged as a means to fundamentally transform the service system. The goals of the reform include enhanced cost containment; improved uniformity of service, along with establishment of a basic standard of care; and an increased rate of timely permanency (James Bell Associates, 2000).

Implementation of Privatization

Kansas adopted a "lead agency model" in which the public agency contracts with private providers to assume responsibility for coordinating and providing services for a defined group of children and families (U.S. GAO, 1998). In Kansas, separate contracts are established in the five regions of the state. Within each region, private agencies bid for single contracts in three program areas: family preservation, foster care and adoption. Originally, in 1997, five different contractors provided family preservation services, three provided foster care and one contractor provided adoption services statewide. An open competitive bidding process occurs every four years. As of July 1, 2000, newly negotiated contracts changed foster care contractors in three regions and family preservation providers in two regions along with establishing a new statewide adoption provider.

Managed Care Features of the System

As originally implemented, contracts with the private providers included a case rate paid in four installments depending upon a child's movement through the system. Case rates are expected to cover the entire operation of the out-of-home-system from shelter to the recruitment of foster parents, regardless of actual costs (U.S. GAO, 1998). Thus, agencies faced a strong financial incentive to find permanent homes for children whether through reunification or adoption (McDonald, Berry, Patterson, & Scott, 2000). Aligning fiscal incentives with permanency goals is one of potential advantages of managed care in child welfare (Feild, 1996; Eggers, 1997; Petr & Johnson, 1998). Yet this arrangement may tempt agencies to under serve children and families to contain costs. To balance this incentive, public agencies establish stringent performance standards to ensure agency accountability (GAO, 1998). In Kansas, for example, outcome goals in foster care include safety from maltreatment, a minimal number of placements and timely reunification. In addition, private provider agencies remain fiscally responsible for children who were placed in their care for 12 months post-case closure.

An Evolving System

The structure of the child welfare system in Kansas continues to evolve in response to unintended consequences as well as the larger context of federal policy changes in child welfare. Flawed assumptions and insufficient planning led to the need for refinement during the initial implementation process (KAC, 1998). Since the advent of privatization, an underestimation of costs and inadequate funding present a challenge to the private agencies (James Bell Associates, 2000). Costs were 65% higher than originally estimated for foster care and 13.5% higher than anticipated for adoption (Kansas Department of Social and Rehabilitation Services, 1999). Fiscal problems led to a special appropriation passed by state legislature in 1999 as well as other tinkering with structure of contracts. The state also determined that original performance standards were unrealistic and worked with providers to establish more sensible goals (U.S. GAO, 1998). Ongoing refinement of outcome measures occurs regularly. In July 2000, with the change in contractors, the state initiated major program modifications, including a new funding method, additional performance measures, and more stringent referral criteria (James Bell Associates, 2000). Most significantly, contracts will no longer be based on case rates but instead utilize a "time in care" payment method in which agencies are paid a monthly capitated amount per child on their caseload, a significant departure from the original assumptions of managed care.

The Impact of Privatized Managed Care on the Child Welfare Workforce

Adopting a model based on managed care principles can have major implications for child welfare personnel (Drissel, 1997). The few studies of privatization and managed care in child welfare focus on the development of fiscal mechanisms and management concerns with only passing acknowledgement of workforce and training issues (Drissel, 1997; Scallet, Brach & Steel, 1997). When staffing is mentioned in relation to privatization and managed care in child welfare, it is usually in regard to public agency issues, such as downsizing and retention (Drissel, 1997; Scallet, Brach & Steel, 1997).

In a notable exception, a 1998 U.S. GAO report outlines new responsibilities for private agencies involved with the implementation of managed care in child welfare. These tasks include hiring, training and retaining qualified case management staff; complying with federal and state administrative requirements, including paperwork; and managing a network of service providers.

Recruitment and Retention of Qualified Workers

Privatization in Kansas resulted in an influx of new workers with little or no child welfare experience. Agencies who were awarded contracts to provide child welfare services expanded as much as three times their original size during the 4 month shift to a privatized system. Providers struggled with recruitment because of shortages of qualified workers in the job market (James Bell Associates, 2000). Initially, it was thought that state child welfare staff would be a primary source for new hires by the private sector. As it happened, most state child welfare personnel remained in their current positions, transferred to other state agencies or opted for early retirement (KAC, 1998). Thus, many new workers were young and inexperienced in child welfare (KAC, 1998, James Bell Associates, 2000). New workers providing the majority of child welfare services potentially affect collateral systems, including the court and mental health systems.

An increase in the number of children coming into state custody in Kansas (KAC, 1998) exacerbated the staffing crisis. After relinquishing responsibility for service provision, public agency workers had more time to investigate alleged abuse and neglect. Feild (1996) cautions that "gatekeepers" in managed care systems that lack day-to-day responsibilities for case management have less incentive to screen out cases. The implication of increasing the number of cases that the system is responsible for could result in increased caseloads, crisis-driven practice and possible delays in permanency.

During the first two years of privatization, staff turnover approached 50% for some agencies (January Scott, personal communication, June 20, 2000). Even now, private provider agencies have urgent and constant need to hire more staff. While the initial surge in foster care has most recently leveled off, the demand for family preservation services exceeded projections by 24% and adoption referrals increased 37% in 1999 (James Bell Associates, 2000).

Factors that are linked to public sector child welfare worker turnover are also inherent in the Kansas system, including high stress, frustration with system, lack of career advancement opportunities and lack of educational preparation for child welfare work (Gleeson, Smith & Dubois, 1993; CWLA, 1990). In foster care, only one of three agencies provided transition time allowing new workers to carry smaller caseloads while receiving more intensive supervision (James Bell Associates, 2000).

The retention of qualified workers is affected by the policies and procedures involved in a privatized system. Potentially, contracts can change in a region at the beginning of each contract period (every 4 years). Upon the impending loss of their jobs, child welfare workers may simultaneously be engaged in the transfer of cases to and interviewing for jobs at the newly awarded contract agency. Consequently, workers feel a lack of job security as their employment status may change independent of their individual proficiency providing child welfare services.

TRAINING IN A MANAGED CARE PRIVATIZED CHILD WELFARE SYSTEM

Commitment and Support for Training

Under privatization, the state's role has shifted from that of service provider to manager of services. Because the state retains statutory responsibility for children in need of care, it must work closely with the private contractors to monitor outcomes for children and families (KAC, 1998). With ultimate responsibility for the performance of the system, arguably, the state should remain interested in the knowledge and skill-level of the public *and* private child welfare workforce. Highly trained workers contribute to enhanced child safety, fewer lawsuits and better outcomes for children and families (Briar-Lawson, Schmid & Harris, 1997). Skilled workers will increase SRS and judicial confidence in private agency work and may eventually decrease some of the need for considerable oversight and monitoring efforts.

The State of Kansas has demonstrated its commitment to a well-trained child welfare workforce by continuing its long-standing collaboration with the University of Kansas to offer training and technical assistance. This support now extends to private child welfare workers. The state's continued involvement and commitment to in-service training for all workers is critical and potentially combats systems issues related to newness of workers and job security.

Infusing the Strengths Perspective in Training Content

The event of privatization created a need to re-evaluate the content and format of training given the new worker/consumer of training services. Agencies that primarily provided group or shelter services to families found themselves in the business of foster care. Again, the increase in staff, shift in philosophy, and tumultuous system created a crisis-like environment for new and on-going staff. Consequently, training curricula focused on information needed for the new workers. Curricula addressed basic skills and knowledge needed for child welfare training, including risk assessment, case planing, developing relationships with mandated clients and goal setting. In an effort to provide training in a format that is effective for new workers working in a crisis-like environment, one and two day training sessions were altered so that materials could be delivered in 3-4 hour sessions.

University of Kansas training staff became concerned about the preparedness of these workers who were new to the field of child welfare as well as being relatively young professionals in an inherently chaotic system. The training and practice concerns focused on the need for new workers to examine their value systems about parenting, biases about gender, ethnicity, and social class, and familiarity with state statutes and agency policy. The basic training addressing the strengths perspective in child welfare practice provided a framework to view work with child welfare families from an outcomes orientation.

Essentially, through the strengths perspective, clients are viewed as possessing strengths across three categories: qualities, talents, and environmental resources. Training focuses on linking the client's strengths across the three categories with case goal achievement and client outcomes. The identification of strengths and the linkages to associated goals is practiced through the use of case scenarios designed by the training staff *as well as* case plans brought to training sessions by participants. This experiential learning allows trainers to assist workers to use the strengths perspective while workers discover tools for client success.

Basic child welfare training for caseworkers and family support workers (who provide transportation and supervise visitation) is the foundation of the curricula. Over time the skill building and learning needs of child welfare professionals span multiple skill levels. The need for basic training continues to be a demand because of high turnover rates and changes in the contractors in various regions. Consequently, the University of Kansas training menu includes basic topics covering issues such as professionalism, boundaries, making the most of visitations, engaging families in the helping process, and managing family crisis.

The University of Kansas training team works closely with private provider agencies to identify on-going training needs. This process of working with management and supervisors is identified as "technical assistance." Through technical assistance, advanced training topics are developed to meet the needs of each agency. The training needs of the agencies vary because of unique relationships between child welfare workers, court personnel, state case monitors and the private child welfare workers, and the geographical location of each region. As a result of technical assistance, training are identified and needs are addressed through various approaches, including developing new training delivered by University of Kansas training team, identifying experts in the community to deliver training for specialized topics, and utilizing national experts for consultation and training in large venues.

The final component of the private provider training curricula is the transfer of learning from the training room to the field. Ultimately, the goal of training is to improve client outcomes. Utilization of "lessons" learned in training requires a change of behavior from "trainee" workers to affect client outcomes. Upon completion of training, trainees must adopt, alter, or eliminate behaviors, skills, and knowledge (Rapp & Kapp, 1999). A multitude of barriers can exist that would derail the adoption of skills and knowledge learned in training. In a privatized system, barriers to skill implementation for child welfare line workers can occur at the individual worker, supervisory unit, private agency, state case monitor, state agency, and juvenile court level. Reinforcing behavior change and adoption of new skills requires a dual process of reinforcing learning and working with the obstacles or barriers to new skill implementation.

In an effort to maximize the transfer of skills from the training environment to the field, the University of Kansas developed a transfer of learning protocol. Intrinsic to this protocol is the belief that training is more than a single event. Training includes supervisors prioritizing skills and knowledge needed by their staff, the training itself and follow-up contacts with supervisors and trainees about implementation as well as barriers to new skills and knowledge.

Implementation of the transfer of learning protocol is a multi-year project. Initially, new training evaluation tools that included domains specific to curricula were developed. Training staff, private agency managers, and supervisors were exposed to the principles of transfer of learning as well as their role in facilitating the increased competence of agency personnel.

Training Outcomes

In fiscal year 1999 the University of Kansas trained 1995. Technical assistance was highly utilized. For example, in the first quarter training staff provided 32 technical assistance contacts to a total of 126 contract staff. Assistance addressed the implementation of curricula to the field and addressed topics such as group supervision and improving outcomes utilizing information management.

Training Challenges

There are several unique training challenges that exist in a privatized environment. Significant challenges include: (1) the timing of training relative to new employment, (2) turnover in contracted agencies, and (3) developing partnerships across private and public agencies for excellence in child welfare practice.

New employees with little experience in child welfare have a myriad of training needs when faced with their first child welfare client. The high worker turnover and the potential influx of new workers following the newly awarded contracts complicate the timing of training delivery. While most agencies encourage participation, and at times mandate participation, training is delivered based on the overall needs of the region. New workers working with a child welfare case for the first time may be required to provide services to a family without any or a minimal orientation to the professional work of child welfare agencies.

The partnership among the public agency, private provider, and University of Kansas training team makes training available. However, participation in an orientation to the skills, tasks and responsibilities of professional work in child welfare does not necessarily occur before workers are faced with clients. In focus groups, some private agency case managers report that their orientation consisted of talking with the burned-out worker leaving their new position (Friesen, 1998). Funds for or the expectation that each private agency will provide a professional orientation is not encouraged or reinforced contractually. Current contracts do not include start-up dollars for training (U.S. GAO, 1998). In this climate, some agencies view training as provided primarily by organizations outside their agency.

The second training challenge is a result of the bidding process for new contracts (occurring approximately every four years). As "old" providers losing new contracts continue to deliver foster care services, the commitment to training for workers facing unemployment is potentially compromised. In addition, new agencies addressing issues related to establishing foster care services for the first time, including designing protocols for transfer of cases from previous providers, developing mechanisms for data collection on client outcomes, creating relationships with foster parents, and interviewing and hiring of new staff (to name a few). The complex issues related to creating or expanding an organization may delay the agency's commitment to or identifying and addressing the staff training needs. The lack of training and disruption in each region potentially compromises the quality of services received by vulnerable children and families.

The third and final challenge in a privatized environment is the development of partnerships and access to federal funds for inventive approaches and training child welfare. With the advent of privatization, all regions are served by a separate agency with unique policies, philosophies, organizational structures, and monitoring systems. Partnering for the development of innovative statewide practice requires the involvement of at least seven organizations (5 private providers, the state agency, and the university). Potential problems exist among the partners in obtaining agreement about the needs of any one sub-population. For instance, while the private provider agencies may be interested in developing innovative practice to improve outcomes for children aging out of the foster care system, the state agency may have other priorities. The state agency's involvement in acquiring funding or developing pilot projects may be reduced based on a variety of issues. These issues include the state's belief about the needs of the child welfare system, state concerns about developing equitable relationships across private provider agencies, and workload issues related to the review, renewing, and loss of private child welfare contracts. In addition, each private provider agency potentially struggles with partnerships that include agencies competing within their region at the next funding cycle. These internal state issues coupled with federal restrictions may inhibit the partnering and financial support of innovated services in a privatized environment.

CONCLUSION

The state of Kansas offers a unique opportunity to learn about the effects of a privatized system designed to improve service for child welfare clients. While Kansas has arguably made the most ambitious shift in service delivery, reportedly 29 states (59%) have one or more "managed care" initiatives planned or underway (McCullough & Schmitt, 2000). While state and private agencies continue to adapt to the intended and unintended results of privatization, the university, private and state agency partnerships provide the foundation for examining, improving, and adapting professional child welfare practice in an evolving system of service delivery.

REFERENCES

Albers, E., Reilly, T. & Rittner, B. (1993). Children in foster care: Possible factors affecting permanency planning. *Child and Adolescent Social Work Journal, 10* (4), 329-341.

Briar-Lawson, K., Schmid, D. & Harris, N. (1997). Improving training, education and practice agendas in public child welfare. *Public Welfare,* 5-7.

Child Welfare League of America. (1990). *Florida Recruitment and Retention Study.* Washington, D.C.: Author.

Dhopper, S. S., Royse, D. D. & Wolfe, L. C. (1990). Does social work education make a difference? *Social Work, 35* (1), 57-61.

Drissel, A. B. (1997). *Managed care and children and family services: A guide for state and local officials.* Baltimore, MD: Annie E. Casey Foundation.

Eggers, W. D. (1997). There's no place like home. *Policy Review, 83,* 43-47.

Feild, T. (1996). Managed care and child welfare: Will it work? *Public Welfare, 54* (3), 4-10.

Friesen, L. D. (1998). *A study of case management in child welfare.* Newton, KS: Bethel College.

Gleeson, J. P., Smith, J. H., & Dubois, A. C. (1993). Developing child welfare practitioners: Avoiding the single-solution seduction. *Administration in Social Work, 17* (3), 21-37.

James Bell Associates. (2000). *External evaluation of the Kansas child welfare system: Year end report (January-December 1999).* Arlington, VA: Author.

Kansas Action for Children, Inc. (1998). *Privatization of child welfare services in Kansas: A child advocacy perspective.* Topeka, KS: Author.

Kansas Department of Social and Rehabilitation Services. (April 1999). *Foster care and adoption cost analysis for children and family services–Final report.* Topeka, KS: Author.

McCullough, C. & Schmitt, B. (2000). Managed care & privatization: Results of a national survey. *Children and Youth Services Review, 22* (2), 117-126.

McDonald, T. P., Berry, M., Patterson, E. & Scott, D. (2000). Adoption trends in Kansas: Managing outcomes or managing care? *Children and Youth Services Review, 22* (2), 161-174.

Olsen, L. & Holmes, W. (1982). Education child welfare workers: The effects of professional training on service delivery. *Journal of Education for Social Work, 18* (1), 94-102.

Petr, C. G. & Johnson, I. C. (1999). Privatization of foster care in Kansas: A cautionary tale. *Social Work, 44* (3), 263-267.

Rapp, C. A. & Kapp, S. A. (1999, March). *Evaluating training: Dilemmas and proposals.* Paper presented at the Child Welfare Training Grantees Meeting, Washington, D.C.

Scallet, L., Brach, C. & Steel, E. (Eds.). (1997). *Managed care: Challenges for children and family services.* Baltimore, MD: Annie E. Casey Foundation.

U.S. Government Accounting Office. (1998). Child welfare: Early experiences implementing a managed care approach. GAO/HEHS-99-8. Washington D.C.: Author.

Evaluating Federally-Funded Child Welfare Training Partnerships: A Worthwhile Challenge

Brenda D. Smith, PhD

SUMMARY. This article assesses the state of evaluation research on federally-funded child welfare training, including both Section 426 and Title IV-E partnerships. The article discusses the need for stronger evaluations of child welfare training and describes some factors which may have impeded past evaluation efforts. It recommends strengthening evaluations of federally-funded child welfare training through well-targeted questions, strong research designs, strong research methods, innovative methods, and theory-driven studies. The article concludes by promoting the development of child welfare research and training centers. *[Article copies available for a fee from The Haworth Document Delivery Service: 1-800-HAWORTH. E-mail address: <getinfo@haworthpressinc.com> Website: <http://www.HaworthPress.com> © 2002 by The Haworth Press, Inc. All rights reserved.]*

KEYWORDS. Child welfare training, evaluation research, social work education

INTRODUCTION

Recognized as important for at least 40 years (see Zlotnik, 2002), effective child welfare training is as vitally needed as ever. New policies, such as the

---

Brenda D. Smith is Assistant Professor in the School of Social Welfare, University at Albany, State University of New York.

[Haworth co-indexing entry note]: "Evaluating Federally-Funded Child Welfare Training Partnerships: A Worthwhile Challenge." Smith, Brenda D. Co-published simultaneously in *Journal of Health & Social Policy* (The Haworth Press, Inc.) Vol. 15, No. 3/4, 2002, pp. 189-201; and: *Evaluation Research in Child Welfare: Improving Outcomes Through University-Public Agency Partnerships* (ed: Katharine Briar-Lawson, and Joan Levy Zlotnik) The Haworth Press, Inc., 2002, pp. 189-201. Single or multiple copies of this article are available for a fee from The Haworth Document Delivery Service [1-800-HAWORTH, 9:00 a.m. - 5:00 p.m. (EST). E-mail address: getinfo@haworthpressinc.com].

Adoption and Safe Families Act, intensify the need to provide quality services in shortened time frames; the needs of child welfare clients are increasingly complex; and specialized skills are increasingly needed in child welfare practice (see Tracy & Pine, 2000). These important needs coincide with a dramatic increase in federal spending on child welfare training partnerships (see Zlotnik, this issue). These combined factors–important needs for effective practice plus dramatically increased training efforts–underscore the importance of an evaluation agenda. We need to understand the effects of child welfare training partnerships, demonstrate their effects, and learn how to maximize their effectiveness.

The articles collected in this volume constitute evidence of several local efforts to evaluate federally-funded child welfare training partnerships. The articles address some key questions related to: recruitment and retention of child welfare staff, differentiation of roles between MSW and BSW practitioners, and the consequences of deprofessionalization in child welfare practice. The articles convey exciting training and evaluation activity.

This article assesses the state of evaluation research on federally-funded child welfare training, including both Section 426 and Title IV-E partnerships. After describing the need for evaluation research, and considering factors which may have impeded past evaluation efforts, the author presents a list of recommendations to strengthen the body of evaluation research on child welfare training partnerships. The author concludes by proposing a way to promote and strengthen evaluation of child welfare training through child welfare research and training centers.

THE NEED FOR EVALUATION STUDIES

The federal commitment to child welfare training reflects perceptions that (1) child welfare agencies need more highly trained staff; and, (2) staff with BSW and MSW degrees, especially BSWs and MSWs with enhanced child welfare training, will improve child welfare services. Such perceptions rest, in part, on a relatively small, yet often-cited, body of studies. Studies have found that child welfare staff with BSW and MSW degrees can be more effective in promoting desired child welfare outcomes (Albers, Reilly, & Rittner, 1993; Dhooper, Royse, & Black, 1990); MSW degrees are associated with better performance in social service work (Booz-Allen & Hamilton, 1987); and, education that includes training in child welfare is associated with longer job retention (CWLA, 1992).

Whereas such research provides a basis for believing that child welfare training can improve child welfare services, existing research varies in the extent to which it can be translated across practice settings, and it leaves a host of unanswered questions. For example, studies of child welfare job acquisition and retention among 426 and IV-E-funded trainees have widely ranging findings. Whereas one study found that 59 percent of trainees obtained child welfare jobs following graduation (Vinokur-Kaplan, 1987), another study found that 93 percent of trainees retained child welfare jobs 4-7 years after their contracted time commitment (Robin & Hollister, 2002). We lack descriptive data on social work students who have benefitted from Section 426 or Title IV-E funding. And we lack descriptive data on the impact of trainees in child welfare agencies, including the average child welfare job tenure of trainees. We need additional research and, especially, additional strong evaluation studies of training partnerships.

PURPOSES OF EVALUATION STUDIES

Evaluation studies serve two primary purposes: they demonstrate effectiveness and they inform stakeholders of ways to increase effectiveness. Attention generally focuses on the need to demonstrate effectiveness. In the case of federally-funded child welfare training, evaluations demonstrate to the federal funding source, universities, schools of social work, child welfare agencies, and the trainees, all of which have invested considerable effort into their success, that the investments are worthwhile. These stakeholders want to see that the considerable investment in child welfare training actually produces well-trained and effective child welfare practitioners.

Evaluations also serve an important role when they inform stakeholders of ways to increase program effectiveness. In the case of federally-funded child welfare training, evaluations might help university and agency partners understand conditions under which the training investments are most effective, and they might suggest ways training efforts could be modified to have a stronger impact on child welfare practice. The demonstration purpose is often associated with "outcome" evaluations, and the informing purpose is often associated with "process" evaluations. However, outcome studies can serve an informing purpose too. For example, when a federal evaluation of Section 426 training programs concluded that "there is little evidence that they respond to the operating needs of state child welfare programs," the specifications of the training grants were modified to encourage involvement of state agencies (Vinokur-Kaplan, 1987).

Many of the studies included in this issue constitute examples of studies which demonstrate effectiveness and/or inform about ways to increase training partnership effectiveness. Among studies that demonstrate effectiveness, several of the studies in this issue assess job retention among Title IV-E and Section 426 trainees. Studies from Minnesota (Robin & Hollister, 2002) and California (Dickinson & Perry, 2002) focus on job retention past the contracted time commitment. The Minnesota study found that 4-7 years after graduation, 93 percent of trainees were still employed in child welfare. The California study found that 3-6 months after completing the contracted commitment, at least 78 percent and up to 88 percent of trainees were still working in child welfare. Another California study (Jones, 2002) reports that 4-5 years after graduation, or about 2-3 years after completing a contracted time commitment, 69 percent of trainees were still employed in child welfare. To assess the extent to which trainees attained leadership positions and made contributions to the field, the same Minnesota study describes trainee's positions and responsibilities. A Louisiana study (Gansle & Ellett, 2002) assesses whether Title IV-E trainees have higher levels of child welfare knowledge than non-trainees both before and after training.

Among studies which inform stakeholders of ways to increase effectiveness, the Minnesota study (Dickinson & Perry, 2002) points to workplace characteristics which influence former trainee's likelihood of staying in child welfare. The evaluators found that the likelihood of staying in child welfare is related to workplace factors such as: time spent on court related activities, perception of supervisor's availability and supportiveness, and opportunities for growth contributing to job satisfaction. Such findings point to the potentially important organizational and workplace factors which may affect the success of child welfare training. Future evaluation studies should further explore these issues. The effects of organizational and workplace characteristics on the success of child welfare staff have been reported in a variety of studies (Glisson & Himmelgarn, 1999; Rycraft, 1994).

In sum, evaluations of child welfare training can both demonstrate effectiveness and provide information on how to increase training effectiveness. Studies such as those included in this issue have begun to serve both purposes. Yet, these purposes should be pursued on a broader scale, involve more partnerships, and use more rigorous research methods.

WHY AREN'T THERE MORE EVALUATION STUDIES?

Given the considerable investment in child welfare training, it is somewhat surprising that we have not seen more evaluation studies as schools strive to demonstrate the value of training dollars. If schools, agencies and trainees truly value the training dollars and see their benefits, what can explain the limited number of studies? Why aren't more partnerships embracing evaluation opportunities?

The minimal evaluation effort could be partly explained by timing. Although Section 426 has funded child welfare training for almost 40 years, and Title IV-E for about 20 years, the training effort has increased considerably only in the last 10 years. Many of the training partnerships are fairly new; considerable training efforts are just beginning. Thus, evaluation opportunities are growing and it is likely that more evaluation studies will emerge in the near future. It is also likely that evaluation studies have been conducted, but not published. This journal issue may indicate the beginning of a growing effort to conduct and publish evaluation studies.

Still, part of the explanation for the minimal evidence of evaluation studies could rest in attitudes toward evaluation research. Whereas demonstrating effectiveness is a key evaluation goal, it is possible that stakeholders in some training partnerships do not embrace evaluation efforts. While key players may see training effects themselves, they may not be persuaded of the need to demonstrate the effects to others. After all, why should partnership members want to invest considerable effort and time to demonstrate what they already know? Evaluations require time and money resources that might otherwise be devoted to the training effort itself. What's more, evaluation research is often associated with politics (see Rubin & Babbie, 1997). Partnership members may have observed past evaluation efforts in which negative evaluation findings were buried or reinterpreted to meet politically acceptable standards. In this context, evaluation might be viewed as an unfortunate and burdensome requirement, rather than a means to obtain helpful information.

A related reason for the surprisingly few published evaluation studies, or a general failure to embrace evaluation efforts, may be that good, useful, evaluation studies are difficult to conduct. Producing strong evaluation research which can clearly demonstrate program effects involves substantial challenges. Educators or agency staff may "know" that child welfare training has positive effects, or they may "see" such effects, but the difficulty and complexity in convincingly demonstrating such effects can be quite daunting. This is especially true in a context characterized by vague and ambiguous outcomes.

If attitudes toward evaluation research are hindering evaluation efforts, we may need conversations among university-based educators and evaluators, agency staff, and trainees about the usefulness of evaluation. Such conversations might address topics such as: the purposes served by evaluation, the features which distinguish useful from non-useful evaluations, and ways to make evaluations more useful. Following such conversations, perhaps some training partners would choose to refine their evaluation objectives. For example, even stakeholders who are convinced of a partnership's effectiveness might see value in evaluations which address questions related to *increasing* training effectiveness. Rather than seeing the evaluation findings as something needed to prove effectiveness to others, some stakeholders might consider ways in which evaluation data can be helpful to *insiders*. Likewise, stakeholders who are daunted by the challenges involved in conducting strong and convincing evaluations, might be encouraged through other's examples or through opportunities for consultation in evaluation design and methods.

Practitioners and researchers alike may question the usefulness of evaluation research. Practitioners can see it as an interruption, as a distraction from their main purpose, or as checking up. Researchers can see it as back bench work or as the least glamorous type of research. Such perceptions can create a double bind. Stakeholders will not be committed to evaluation studies if they do not consider the studies useful. Yet, studies are not likely to be useful unless stakeholders are first committed to them. The following section includes suggestions for strengthening the base of evaluation studies of federally-funded child welfare training so that the evaluations might become more useful.

STEPS TOWARD STRONG, USEFUL, VITAL EVALUATION STUDIES

We need more good evaluation studies of federally-funded child welfare training. Useful evaluation studies are characterized by: well-targeted questions, strong research designs, strong research methods, innovative methods, and theory-driven studies.

Well-Targeted Questions

To be useful, outcome evaluations must focus on outcomes which are neither too rudimentary nor too distant from the program to show an effect. For child welfare training, one might imagine a hierarchy of outcomes: completing training; demonstrating increased child welfare knowledge and/or skill; completing a contracted time commitment; maintaining public child welfare employment past a contracted time commitment; performing well in public child welfare positions; and improving child and family client outcomes. The most useful and intriguing evaluations will go beyond demonstrating that trainees completed training; such information can be documented in a statistical tracking report. At the same time, the most useful and intriguing evaluations will not seek to demonstrate aggregate effects in complex outcomes such as a community's child placement rate or adoption rate. We might expect child welfare training to affect child welfare practice and, consequently, to affect families and communities, but at an aggregate level, the influence of training is likely to be overpowered by the many other factors influencing families and communities. Such outcomes might be explored qualitatively in close-up exploratory studies of child welfare practice, however, as discussed below.

Several of the articles in this issue address outcomes in the middle range. Examples of middle-range questions related to demonstrating training effectiveness that are addressed by the studies in this issue, and which might be addressed by other partnerships include: What proportion of federally-funded child welfare trainees work in child welfare following graduation? What proportion of trainees exceed their contracted time commitment? To what extent have child welfare trainees provided leadership or made special contributions to the field of child welfare (Robin & Hollister, 2002)? What is the average tenure of trainees in child welfare jobs (Jones, 2002)? How do funded trainees compare to other social work students in the level of pre and post training child welfare knowledge (Gansle & Ellett, 2002)? How do trainees compare to other child welfare staff of similar experience in their supervisor-assessed performance (Brown, Chavkin & Peterson, 2002)? How do trainees assess their knowledge and capacity to use the knowledge once they enter child welfare practice (Wehrmann, Shin, & Poertner, 2002)?

Just as outcome evaluations might focus on intriguing middle-range questions, process evaluations might go beyond documenting curriculum content, implementation timelines, and training processes. Examples of questions related to increasing training effectiveness which are addressed by the studies in this issue, and which might be addressed by other partnerships include: How do trainees who remain or plan to remain in child welfare following their contracted time commitment differ from trainees who leave or plan to leave (Dickinson & Perry, 2002)? What supervisor characteristics best promote trainee's effectiveness (Gansle & Ellett, 2002)? Other questions related to increasing training effectiveness, which other evaluation studies might address include: Do different curricula have different outcomes? Are different curricula more effective with BSW or MSW students? How should BSW training differ from MSW training?

Is training more effective for experienced staff or for new practitioners? How should training curricula differ for trained staff versus new practitioners? What organizational characteristics promote the success of trainees? What can trainees and partnerships do to foster the organizational characteristics which promote success? Posing evaluation questions at the right level is a first step toward addressing useful and intriguing evaluation studies.

Strong Research Designs

Strong research designs also contribute to making evaluation studies useful and intriguing. Evaluators should make efforts to pursue experimental and quasi-experimental designs. Experimental designs would involve random assignment of trainees to alternative conditions. For example, trainees could be randomly assigned to alternative curricula or alternative field experiences. Quasi-experimental designs might involve a control group of non-trainees. A host of interesting comparisons could be made as long as researchers collect sufficient baseline data to control for preexisting differences between a trainee group and control group. For example, trainees could be compared to child welfare practitioners who lack special child welfare training, or who lack social work degrees. Graduates of federally funded child welfare training programs could be compared to graduates of other types of social work education. Graduates of training programs who pursue public child welfare jobs could be compared to graduates who pursue voluntary sector child welfare jobs. Training outcomes in one state could be compared to training outcomes in another state.

Strong evaluation designs are unlikely to result if the evaluation of child welfare training is an afterthought, conducted only to comply with requirements, or attached to the end of a child welfare training program. The implementation of strong evaluation designs usually requires that evaluation become a priority. Evaluation studies need to be planned in conjunction with the training program so that evaluation efforts can begin as students enter training. Such planning would facilitate the use of both experimental and quasi-experimental research designs.

Strong Research Methods

In addition to stronger research designs, useful evaluations would be promoted through the use of more rigorous research methods. Studies would benefit through increased efforts to collect baseline data, through efforts to obtain higher survey response rates and tests of response bias, and through means to obtain larger numbers of study participants.

Baseline data. With long-range research goals in mind, all programs should collect baseline data on funded trainees and comparison groups. Baseline data could be used to assess change over time in knowledge or skill among trainees, to compare pre-existing characteristics of trainees to non-trainees, and to control for the effects of pre-existing characteristics on educational and career outcomes.

Survey response. In addition to collecting baseline data, evaluators conducting surveys of training graduates could take several steps to improve the rigor of their survey research. Evaluators could explain long-term research plans to program participants. Participants could be asked to provide contact persons who are likely to know their whereabouts over time. Such steps could improve survey response rates. Several studies in this issue were hindered by low survey response rates, often due to the lack of current contact information.

In addition, survey researchers should use the baseline data collected from all program trainees to conduct tests for response bias. Tests for response bias would tell us how survey respondents differ from the non-respondents, and would aid in the interpretation of survey results. All studies should obtain data on all program participants to provide the opportunity to test for response bias, especially in the event of low survey response rates.

Larger numbers. Low numbers are a challenging problem faced by many evaluations of training partnerships. If only 5-10 trainees graduate from a particular university each year, evaluators focusing only on that program will face problems with low numbers. Some current evaluations may contain Type II error because they lack the sample sizes to have adequate statistical power to detect differences between groups. Evaluators should conduct power analyses to assess the sample sizes needed to detect statistically significant differences. Adequate sample sizes might not be available to address certain explanatory research questions, or to test certain hypotheses. If not, studies should focus on descriptive questions or use other research methods. To increase study numbers, partnerships might consider aggregating program graduates over a period of time or conducting evaluations that combine several partnerships within a state or region. Such efforts would be promoted through development of region-based child welfare research centers discussed below. Larger numbers would enable evaluators to conduct multivariate analysis which could help rule out competing explanations for findings. Several partnerships have reported an association between trainees and certain characteristics, including age, race, and prior child welfare experience. Such differences among trainees could obscure or otherwise confound training effects. Multivariate analyses could help tease out such relationships.

Innovative Research Methods

As the article by Anderson-Butcher, Lawson and Barkdull (2002) demonstrates, innovative research methods, including participatory and qualitative methods, constitute important additions to the evaluation knowledge base. Anderson-Butcher and colleagues describe an effort of four Western states to use collaborative evaluation teams. Collaborative evaluation teams might involve university professors, agency staff, students, community members and even child welfare clients. Whereas schools of social work have an important perspective on the training programs and the criteria for success, agency staff, community members, trainees and clients bring other perspectives, including, perhaps, other conceptual frameworks for how training in child welfare could improve child welfare services. Trainee students, graduates, agency personnel and community members could be involved in the design and implementation of evaluation studies, rather than consulted only as respondents in evaluation studies.

Due to the multitude of factors that affect child welfare outcomes, training partnerships are not likely to demonstrate measurable effects upon outcomes such as a locality's foster care placement rates, reunification rates or adoption rates. Yet, qualitative studies, such as ethnographies, might explore how child welfare training is used by practitioners in communities. In-depth studies of child welfare workers might document how training knowledge is applied, or how training knowledge affects practice, and consequently, how it affects a particular child's or family's outcomes. Qualitative studies might also document the ways agencies change as trainees become part of the staff. Such qualitative work might document when, whether, or how increasing numbers of child welfare trainees eventually constitute a critical mass which changes organizational culture (see Hopkins, Murdick, & Rudolph, 1999).

Theory-Driven Studies

The importance of outcome studies should not overshadow the importance of conducting theory-driven studies. Evaluators should avoid producing "black box" assessments of outcome effects without theoretical or conceptual explanations of the processes which produce the effects (see Sherraden, 2000). Under a black box scenario, even if a study produces convincing evidence that a particular training program resulted in desired outcomes, it would be difficult to replicate that success without theory or evidence suggesting how the program was successful. Evaluation studies cannot contribute to a building knowledge base unless it is possible to make comparisons across programs or studies. Thus, studies should reflect a logic model, conceptual framework or theory (see Wright, 1999).

Evaluations should first reflect a conceptual framework which designates relationships between key constructs of child welfare training and desired trainee and practice outcomes. Evaluators should then explain how such relationships link to more general concepts. There is a considerable knowledge base in the transfer of knowledge to practice, adult learning, and organizational characteristics which promote or hinder the capacity to use new knowledge. Evaluation studies of child welfare training could be enhanced substantially by using and building upon such knowledge. For example, the transfer of training model outlined by Wehrmann, Shin and Poertner (2002) clearly defines three levels of factors which affect transfer of training to practice: individual factors, training curriculum factors and organizational factors. If knowledge is most likely to be transferred to practice under certain organizational conditions, evaluators should include measures of such organizational conditions when assessing knowledge transfer. Evaluations reflecting a conceptual framework which links to general concepts will both benefit from prior theory and research and contribute to a building knowledge base.

A SUPPORTIVE STRUCTURE TO BUILD AN EVIDENCE-BASED MOVEMENT

Strong evaluation studies could be promoted, supported and disseminated through national or regional child welfare research centers. These centers could constitute the supportive structure for a data and theory driven movement to improve child welfare training research. In addition to providing a clearinghouse to catalog and share information, building upon the recent training partnerships newsletter, the centers could serve the purposes of evaluation consultation, dissemination assistance, implementation guidance, and collaboration facilitation.

Evaluation consultation. The research centers could provide advice on evaluation design and methods. They could develop some evaluation models for researchers to follow or adapt. In addition, the centers could provide a networking structure to link researchers addressing similar issues. A mentoring system could be developed in which more experienced and successful evaluators assist less experienced evaluators. The centers could link evaluators with consultants in evaluation design, statistics, and qualitative or other innovative methods.

Dissemination assistance. If evaluation findings are disseminated, the benefits of stronger evaluations can extend beyond their local partnerships. Child welfare research centers could provide means to disseminate findings through electronic and conventional means. A mechanism to dissemination evaluation studies could help to enforce the message that the evaluation work is important.

Implementation guidance. Child welfare research centers could assist partnerships in implementing changes suggested by evaluation findings. The centers could recommend curriculum changes, or work with partnerships to implement agency-based changes to promote successful child welfare practice of the child welfare trainees.

Collaboration facilitation. Collaborative evaluation efforts between states or within regions could move beyond the question, "Does child welfare training in our area create the desired outcomes?" Collaborative efforts could support research questions such as: How does training vary in different states? Are different training programs having different types of success? Are different practice environments resulting in better outcomes for trainees? For agencies or child welfare clients?

National leadership is needed for a data and theory driven structure to strengthen child welfare training research. Existing social work and child welfare organizations, including the Institute for the Advancement of Social Work Research (IASWR), the Children's Bureau, the Child Welfare League of America (CWLA), the National Association of Social Workers (NASW), and the Council on Social Work Education (CSWE) might play an initial role in fostering the effort and developing leadership.

CONCLUSION

The articles assembled in this collection convey exciting training and evaluation activity. Yet, against a backdrop which includes multiple university-agency training partnerships, millions of dollars devoted to social work education for child welfare workers, and a large number of trainees prepared for child welfare work, we might expect more evidence of evaluation efforts. We might expect evidence of a nationwide effort to study and document the implementation and outcomes of federally-funded child welfare training.

At this moment, we have both a tremendous need for effective child welfare training and the increasing use of federal funding to provide it. Exciting child welfare training partnerships are in place all around the country. The combination of these factors highlights the responsibility to evaluate and communicate the effects of child welfare training partnerships. This responsibility is not only one of accountability to federal funders, it is one of accountability to the practitioners trained through the partnerships, the agencies participating in the partnerships and, ultimately, the children and families who receive child welfare services. But evaluation efforts do more than demonstrate to these stakeholders that training partnerships can effectively meet their objectives. Evaluation efforts can also produce important information about how partnership efforts can be improved, or how their effectiveness can be increased. Increasing the effectiveness of child welfare training is a worthy objective that we should embrace through improved, expanded, and coordinated evaluation efforts.

REFERENCES

Albers, E., Reilly, T., & Rittner, B. (1993). Children in foster care: Possible factors affecting permanency planning. *Child and Adolescent Social Work Journal*, 10 (4), 329-341.

Anderson-Butcher, D., Lawson, H. & Barkdull, C. (2002). An evaluation of child welfare design teams in four states. *Journal of Health & Social Policy*, 15 (3/4), 131-161.

Booz-Allen & Hamilton, Inc. (1987). The Maryland social services job analysis and personnel qualifications study, executive summary. Baltimore: Maryland Department of Human Resources.

Briar-Lawson, K. & Wisen, M. (1999). Effective partnership models between state agencies, the university, and community service providers. In *Changing Paradigms of Child Welfare Practice: Responding to Opportunities and Challenges.* Washington, DC. U.S. Department of Health and Social Services, Administration on Children, Youth and Families, Children's Bureau.

Brown, J.K., Chavkin, N.F. & Peterson, V. (2002). Tracking process and outcomes results of BSW students' preparation for public child welfare practice: Lessons learned. *Journal of Health & Social Policy,* 15 (3/4), 105-116.

Child Welfare League of America (CWLA). (1992). Staffing the child welfare agency: Recruitment and retention. Washington, DC: Author.

Dhooper, S. S., Royse, D. D., & Wolfe, L. C. (1990). Does social work education make a difference? *Social Work,* 35, 57-61.

Dickinson, N.S. & Perry, R.E. (2002). Factors influencing the retention of specially educated public child welfare workers. *Journal of Health & Social Policy,* 15 (3/4), 89-103.

Gansle, K.A. & Ellett, A.J. (2002). Child welfare knowledge transmission, practitioner retention and university-community impact: A study of Title IV-E child welfare training. *Journal of Health & Social Policy,* 15 (3/4), 69-88.

Gleeson, J. P., Smith, J. H., & Dubois, A. C. (1993). Developing child welfare practitioners: Avoiding the single-solution seduction. *Administration in Social Work,* 17 (3), 21-37.

Glisson, C. & Hemmelgarn, A. (1998). The effects of organizational climate and interorganizational coordination on the quality and outcomes of children's service systems. *Child Abuse and Neglect,* 22 (5), 401-421.

Hopkins, K. M., Mudrick, N. R., & Rudolph, C. S. (1999). Impact of university/agency partnerships in child welfare on organizations, workers, and work activities. *Child Welfare,* 78 (6), 749-773.

Jones, L. (2002). A follow-up of a title IV-E program's graduates' retention rates in a public child welfare agency. *Journal of Health & Social Policy,* 15 (3/4), 39-51.

Robin, S.C. & Hollister, C.D. (2002). Career paths and contributions of four cohorts of IV-E funded MSW child welfare graduates. *Journal of Health & Social Policy,* 15 (3/4), 53-67.

Rose, S. J. (1999). Educating adult learners for child welfare practice: The Wisconsin experience with Title IV-E. *Journal of Teaching in Social Work,* 18 (1/2), 169-183.

Rubin, A. & Babbie, E. (1997). *Research Methods for Social Work, Third Edition.* Pacific Grove, CA: Brooks/Cole Publishing Company.

Rycraft, J. R. (1994). The party isn't over: The agency role in the retention of public child welfare caseworkers. *Social Work,* 39 (1), 75-80.

Sherraden, M. (2000). Asking questions well: The role of theory in applied social research. *Proceedings of the Twelfth National Symposium on Doctoral Research in Social Work.* Columbus, Ohio: Ohio State University College of Social Work.

Tracy, E. M. & Pine, B. A. (2000). Child welfare education and training: Future trends and influences. *Child Welfare,* 79 (1), 93-113.

Vinokur-Kaplan, D. (1987). Where did they go? A national follow-up of child welfare trainees. *Child Welfare,* 66 (5), 411-421.

Wehrmann, K. C., Shin, H., & Poertner, J. (2002). Transfer of training: An evaluation study. *Journal of Health & Social Policy,* 15 (3/4), 23-37.

Wright, L. (1999). Documenting project outcomes helps build knowledge base. *Partnerships for Child Welfare,* December 1999. Council on Social Work Education.

Zlotnik, J.L. (2002). Preparing social workers for child welfare practice: Lessons from an historical review of the literature. *Journal of Health & Social Policy,* 15 (3/4), 5-21.

Index